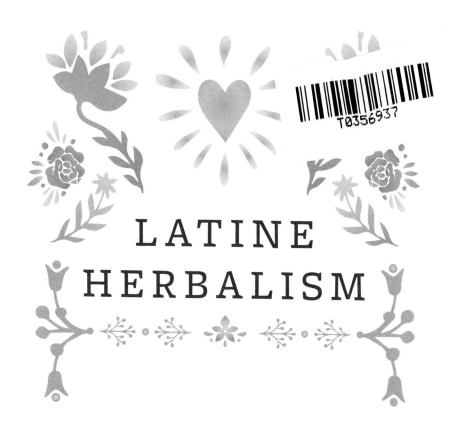

LATINE
HERBALISM

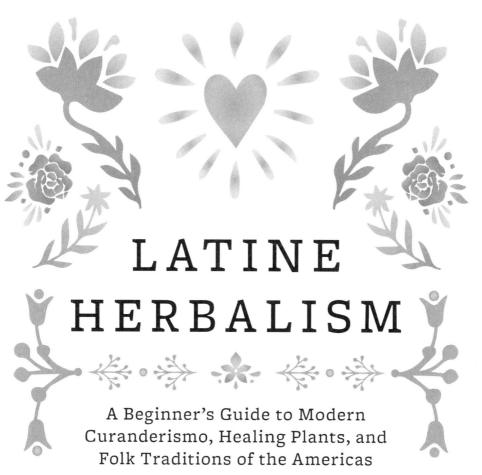

LATINE
HERBALISM

A Beginner's Guide to Modern
Curanderismo, Healing Plants, and
Folk Traditions of the Americas

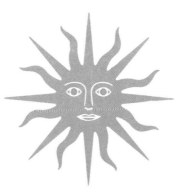

IOSELLEV CASTAÑEDA

Published by:
ULYSSES PRESS
32 Court Street, Suite #2109
Brooklyn, NY 11201
www.ulyssespress.com

ISBN: 978-1-64604-762-8
Library of Congress Control Number: 2024945008

Printed in the United States
10 9 8 7 6 5 4 3 2 1

Acquisitions editor: Claire Sielaff
Project editor: Renee Rutledge
Managing editor: Claire Chun
Editor: Mary Barbosa
Front cover design: Raquel Castro
Shutterstock.com images: cover based on artwork by © Yamurchik, © Vector street, © RedKoala; interior pages 6, 29, 49, 113 © Epine; page 27 © Babich Alexander; page 28 mason jar © Mara Fribus, Boston round bottle © chelovector, kettle © Marina Levshina; page 48 © Havryliuk-Kharzhevska; pages 53, 56, 91 © SpicyTruffel; page 65 © DiviArts; page 66 © Qualit Design; page 77 © Morning Glory; page 81 © Sopelkin; pages 82, 131, 153, 162 © Foxyliam; page 93 © GoodStudio; page 98 © Istry Istry

NOTE TO READERS: This book has been written and published strictly for informational and educational purposes only. It is not intended to serve as medical advice or to be any form of medical treatment. You should always consult your physician before altering or changing any aspect of your medical treatment and/or undertaking a diet regimen. Do not stop or change any prescription medications without the guidance and advice of your physician. Any use of the information in this book is made on the reader's good judgment after consulting with his or her physician and is the reader's sole responsibility. This book is not intended to diagnose or treat any medical condition and is not a substitute for a physician. This book is independently authored and published and no sponsorship or endorsement of this book by, and no affiliation with, any trademarked brands or other products mentioned within is claimed or suggested. All trademarks that appear in ingredient lists and elsewhere in this book belong to their respective owners and are used here for informational purposes only. The author and publisher encourage readers to patronize the brands mentioned in this book.

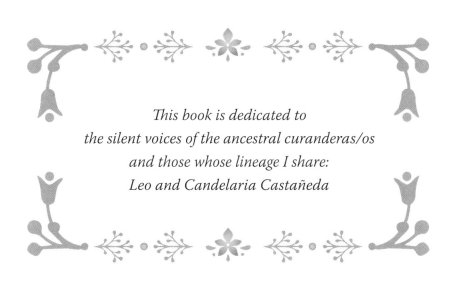

This book is dedicated to
the silent voices of the ancestral curanderas/os
and those whose lineage I share:
Leo and Candelaria Castañeda

CONTENTS

CHAPTER 1

INTRODUCTION & ORGANIZATION

¡BIENVENIDXS!

In December 2015, I created a "book" folder on my laptop to start collecting recipes, notes, observations, and the like for the possibility of writing a book someday. It has taken ten years for this book to manifest. Along the way, I have learned and integrated various teachings that support the *remedios y rituales* (remedies and rituals) sections of this book. Latine herbalism today can encompass many cultures and myriad ways to address folk healing. With this book, I share folk remedies from my own cultural heritage of Mexican-Cuban ancestry. Some of what I learned came via living tradition—folk remedies used in daily life taught to me by my mother and father—while other teachings stemmed from Western herbalist teachers.

Writing this book was a quest in itself. There were many things I wanted to share, and some things I knew intuitively that no book had yet presented. Much about Latine herbalism is taught orally and varies depending on family tradition or the culture from which it derives. My objective in putting these chapters together was neither to create an encyclopedia nor to detail traditional *curanderismo*. In truth, I merely want to share the knowledge of Latine herbalism for today's modern way of life. I aim to include easily found herbs and streamlined applications for modern-day ailments, supporting contemporary views of energy and vibration with rituals that have been passed down from my ancestral lines, while encouraging you to create your own.

It is important to mention that Latine herbalism concepts are for anyone who has an appreciation for Latine communities and culture. We are a warm people who are always happy to include others in our activities, festivities, and way of life. We include everyone! *Donde come uno, comen dos.* My friend and someone I consider a second mother, Gladys Perez, always said this to me. It translates to, "Where one person eats, two people can eat." It is a very true and very accurate description of our generosity as a culture, regardless of which Latin American country we are from. You are all invited to my table to share in rituals, remedies, and stories as I share in this book.

A MODERN CURANDERA

As a Mexican-Cuban-American woman, my point of view is influenced by the heritage I hold and my lived experience. I cannot separate the teachings of my family from those of my mentors, as they all flow through me and manifest uniquely. The information I share here is ultimately filtered through both. You will find in this book a beautiful braid of knowledge weaving together my Mexican maternal line, my Cuban paternal line, and the Western line of European knowledge I have chosen to study.

My personal journey with folk herbalism began in my twenties with the use of herbs to help me manage my busy life as a fashion designer living in NYC—one in which I wanted to work fourteen-hour days, maintain a weekend side business, and still have time for friends, family, a relationship, travel, fun, and higher education. At that time, I was convinced I could do it all.

I would drink a lavender-chamomile blend tea at bedtime from a known commercial tea maker to relax my body, and a *guaraná*-infused drink to pep me up when I needed to focus or burn through a deadline. But it was later, in my thirties, that I learned how to use herbs for overall well-being. This was when I realized that, during my childhood, my family had used herbs along with other rituals to combat a variety of ailments. This is also when I recognized that today's illnesses, worries, and "dis-ease" are not the same as those of our grandparents or even our parents.

An interest in meditation led, in my late twenties, to becoming a certified yoga instructor. In the modality and philosophy of yoga, I found a synergistic approach to wellness. My studies in an NYC ashram lasted five years, and I loved every minute. Meditating calmed my mind, focused my energy, and allowed me to see the world from a different perspective. Even now, twenty-one years later, I continue a solid meditation practice. Meditation with correct instruction—including mantras, japa mala (prayer beads), and dedicated guidance—can lead to sustained mental awareness and overall well-being. Substantial research explores the brain's function and the body's response to consistent meditation. Dr. Joe Dispenza, for example, has conducted long-term studies in this area with remarkable results. Through the practice of meditation, I later found myself open and curious about yoga asanas (the physical exercises), Ayurveda (the traditional Hindu system of herbal remedies), and, later on, traditional Western herbalism, the most popular form of herbalism today.

By my thirties, I had studied for a few years with folk herbalists from the NYC area, learning about herb qualities, apothecary preparations, and how to diagnose illnesses and offer supportive remedies. I began to associate the herbs of my childhood with my parents' stories about miraculous herb-induced healings.

Although I never pursued an apprenticeship, eventually, curiosity led me to the doorstep of Julia Graves—master herbalist, classical homeopath, flower essence creator, psychotherapist, and bodyworker. Her teachings on flower essences, along with the supportive principles she shares, opened a door to the understanding of vibration and energy healing. From that moment on, I felt as if a bright light was turned on in my own energy field, and I began to pursue modalities of energetic wellness, feeling as if that was the one missing piece in a puzzle that, until then, I had no idea I was part of. After a year of trials, I settled on the study of traditional Usui Reiki, an alternative, hands-on modality of vibrational and energetic healing. I spent six years practicing and fine-tuning my perception of energy, which led to heightened intuition and a realization that my next step in life was to support others in their healing journey.

After years of studying and practicing other cultures' healing modalities, I began to inquire about the healing practices of my own culture. The remembrance of childhood remedies and rituals came to me in pieces until I actively pursued curanderismo. The rich stories of folk remedies used by my Mexican and Cuban great-grandparents revealed themselves as I read about the Latine healing modality. It was interesting to learn that the curanderismo of the pueblos and small communities in Mexico was different from that practiced in Cuba, the Caribbean islands, and other Latin American countries. The "traditional" version of remedies and rituals shifted according to geographical origin and oral traditions. It was this element of curanderismo that gave me the freedom to incorporate my knowledge of yoga, Ayurveda, folk herbalism, and Reiki into my own alternative healing practice. This interweaving of multicultural knowledge shaped me into a modern-day *curandera* (healer), allowing me to share curanderismo and Latine herbalism with others.

Today's ailments are not the same as those of even twenty years ago. The stress of living a conventional life—in which the priority is on external values such as education, job, house, car, marriage, kids, college tuition, and so on—has given way to ailments that affect our nervous systems and mental states. The global pandemic of 2020 gave many of us time to reflect on our fast-paced lifestyles, and for some, it was a wake-up call to do better and shift priorities to a more mindful and slower-paced life. While many were able to make these changes, many also became aware of the high intensity they were living with but were unable to step out of. With this book, I hope to share how Latine herbalism and modern curanderismo can support you in making small changes for a better life. For those seasoned folk herbalists among you, my wish is that this book will open you to other cultural healing modalities and inspire you to integrate them into your personal practice.

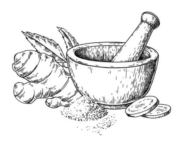

WHAT ARE LATINE HERBALISM AND CURANDERISMO?

Definitions

Curanderismo means "system of healing" in Spanish: *curando*—healing (the act of healing), and *ismo*—system.

Curanderismo today is a blend of Indigenous and European healing. It is believed by many to be a "true" and Indigenous healing modality due to its use throughout Latin America—but it is not. When I first began to educate myself on the topic, I found it difficult to think of curanderismo as a blend of modalities; from my experience, it was a purely Mexican approach to healing. However, as I learned, during colonialism, the Indigenous peoples of Mexico, Central, and South America hid or replaced their gods with the "new gods" to salvage and continue some of their original practices, submerging their ancient ways to avoid persecution. Thus, curanderismo was heavily influenced by Catholic beliefs to appease the colonizers and demonstrate that healing practices were nonthreatening. Religious conversion occurred alongside the preservation of the original divinity and sacred energy of ancestral philosophies, religions, and healing ways. Curanderismo today incorporates remedios y rituales that represent the culmination of centuries of practice.

Early curanderismo was a beautiful example of survival. In addition to maintaining some of the Indigenous ways, it also incorporated new cultural healing modalities introduced by the colonizers, including the Greek philosophy of humors, the modality of cupping, and botanical preparations according to European standards of the day. Latine herbalism sprouts from this tradition of curanderismo. It is the offspring of the system of healing that our grandmothers, great-grandmothers, and ances-tors used to support their families and communities through times of colonialism and migration.

Traditional folk healing methods of many cultures viewed affliction and disease as an imbalance of the mental, emotional, and physical bodies. Similarly, curanderismo focuses on both physical and energetic wellness. The remedios y rituales we will explore in this book offer both physical and energetic healing to support the whole person—in today's terms, it is a *holistic* approach to healing. Let's break down these two different types of healing.

Energy Healing Versus Physical Healing

Energetic healing is used by curanderas/os to address mental and emotional afflictions that sometimes manifest in unfamiliar physical symptoms. Its signature method—the *plática* (a chat, heart-straightening talk, or spiritual consultation)—is a form of psychotherapy in which the curandera/o listens, gives advice, and sometimes proposes herbal remedies to support healing. Yet, the bulk of energetic healing occurs through simple rituals known as *limpias* (energy cleanses). As the name implies, this practice effects an energy cleaning of the vibrational body. Where heavy, stagnant, or unwanted energy is found, it is cleared and released. Traditional limpias include Catholic elements of prayers, saints' candles, and rosaries, along with botanical *barridas* (body sweeps) and *baños* (basin baths). Some of these are part of a religious expression, but as a nonreligious curandera, I offer modern rituals in my practice. These include flower and crystal essences, crystal bowl sound healing, and advanced Reiki protocols. Ailments found in the vibrational body—such as *susto* (fright, shock), *mal de ojo* (evil eye), *maldiciones y traiciones* (curses and betrayals), and *melancolía* (depression, sorrow, grief)—can manifest as mental and emotional afflictions that often inspire people to seek help from a curandera/o.

Physical healing in curanderismo is called for when an individual has a disease rooted in the body. Here, curanderismo offers three specializations—*hueseras/os* (bone and muscle specialists), *yerberas/os* (herbalists), and *parteras/comadronas* (midwives and doulas). These specialties vary by family lineage and are usually learned through apprenticeships. Apprenticeships in curanderismo are lifelong and often reserved for family or important community members.

- **Hueseras/os** are both masseuses and orthopedic healers. They focus on the body and offer support with a plática and work through ailments such as broken bones and muscular issues and pain. They sometimes address energetic afflictions that might bring on physical disease.

- **Yerberas/os** offer herbal support to the body, mind, and energy. They often assume the role of physicians in their communities. Yerberas/os sometimes use physical manipulation of the body via massage and *ventosas* (cupping). They can also conduct lengthy pláticas and use herbs to alleviate mental and emotional afflictions.

- **Parteras/comadronas** are equivalent to today's midwives and doulas. Predominantly women, these curanderas follow strict, lineage-based studies. A young woman may be shown the path to become a partera after she herself gives birth to her first child or by assisting her mother or grandmother in the processes of fertility, childbirth, and childrearing as a child.

Hueseras/os, yerberas/os, and parteras/comadronas practice the modality of opposites, sometimes called the *frio-caliente* (cold-hot) method. Traditional Western Herbalism (TWH) and Traditional European Herbalism, also known as folk herbalism in the USA, follow the modality of opposites as well.

We are learning today about the philosophies of Indigenous peoples in South America, Africa, and Australia, in which humans are not the center of life and Nature is held in the highest regard.

In this ideology, we are part of Nature, and Nature lives in us. This belief system mirrors that of our ancestors when life was lived in tune with Nature, respecting the changing seasons and trusting in the bounty of plants. The controlled environments we live in today—air conditioning, heating, humidifiers, and dehumidifiers—were not part of their daily lives. Toiling over their harvest under the hot sun, sleeping beneath the cool moonbeams, warming their bodies by the fire, and experiencing frigid river and lake waters gave them firsthand experience with Nature. Our ancestors understood inherently that everything—including our bodies—is composed of the elements earth, water, fire, and air. TWH developed from the logic that we can use natural allies in the form of plants and minerals to recalibrate and bring balance to the body and mind when there is affliction or disease. If an element is lacking, we can increase it. If an element is in excess, we can diminish it. Today's Traditional Western Herbalism, a natural system of physical healing developed through trial and error, is a categorized system that applies elemental qualities to herbs and afflictions.

While curanderismo and Latine herbalism are influenced by and sometimes directly reflect TWH principles, they can be practiced more intuitively. Traditionally, set protocols or processes for treating certain afflictions and diseases are inherently known by experienced curanderas/os, who can offer specific remedies and support the work of parteras and hueseras.

In some Central and South American countries, other healing modalities such as divination, faith healing, and hands-on healing are also considered part of curanderismo, making curanderas/os sometimes synonymous with tarot readers and fortune-tellers.

These modalities are not traditional to the curanderismo system in Mexico and the USA, despite many individuals throughout the history of curanderismo having demonstrated these abilities. Traditionally, curanderas/os possess heightened intuition and are able to offer a holistic approach to healing. To learn more about this, I suggest the book *Curandero: Traditional Healers of Mexico and the Southwest* (2017) by Eliseo "Cheo" Torres and Imanol Miranda. Torres is considered the leading scholar and advocate of curanderismo in the USA.

It is interesting to note that Indigenous healers do not call themselves curanderas/os. While they might use Indigenous-language words for "healer" or "light worker," it is important to honor these healers in their preference not to be called hueseras/os, yerberas/os, parteras, or curanderas/os. Their philosophies and healing methods are private and sacred. This is also the case with shamans. I hold much respect for shamans and the shamanic practices and traditions of Peru and the Amazon. Their practices are highly interwoven with the energetic realms, and while they, too, utilize herbs, plants, and pláticas, their approach to healing differs from curanderismo. Although due to the Spanish language some shamans and healers are called curanderas/os and *sanadores* (healers), their practices are different.

Lastly, a long-held belief about curanderas/os is that their ability to support the healing process is measured not by knowledge, expertise, or studies alone but by the enigmatic *don*—the gift of healing. For example, my father used only one herb to support others in their holistic healing. He preferred verbena (Jamaican vervain) and recommended it for all healing capacities, from digestive issues to muscular pain to energetic cleanses.

The beauty of this: it worked for every occasion! I believe that, in these cases, there is a relationship between healer and recipient that is unexplained. The trust and faith in the healer work like mind over matter with unexpected, positive results.

The Five Elements and Four Qualities

Drawing on our ancestors' reverence for the elements, the school of TWH developed a cohesive manner of categorizing the elemental energies into four qualities, also known as the tissue states, in order to identify the condition of the affliction (or "dis-ease"). These qualities help us identify the physical energies of corresponding herbs. The five elements are listed in Chart A from most dense (earth) to least dense (ether), and the four tissue states are identified in Chart B.

Within the modality of opposites, the tissue states help us identify which healing support to use. For example, if the skin is "hot and dry" after a sunburn, we apply an herb that is "cold and damp" to alleviate the discomfort. Recall the cold-hot method mentioned previously; this is the case with all botanical methods in curanderismo and Latine herbalism. Learning the categories and qualities of the elements and tissue states helps streamline the use of botanicals. I will share indigenous and European botanicals along with the physical energies discovered and refined through my personal practice and study with both TWH herbalists and curanderismo.

Chart A: Qualities of the Elements in TWH and Curanderismo/Latine Herbalism

ELEMENT	PRIMARY QUALITY	SECONDARY QUALITY
Earth	Cold	Dry
Water	Wet	Cold
Fire	Hot	Dry
Air	Moist	Hot
Ether	Cool	Moist

Chart B: The Tissue States in TWH and Curanderismo/Latine Herbalism

ELEMENTS BY TISSUE STATE	PRIMARY QUALITY
Dry	Flaky skin
Hot	Red burn
Damp	Sweating during fever
Cold	White/blue color of frost bite

You may ask why TWH receives so much emphasis. Simply put, many of the herbs used in Latine herbalism and curanderismo in the USA and Latin America derive from European roots. Many of the herbs considered traditional in curanderismo, such as chamomile and rosemary, are actually replacements of their indigenous counterparts. Having a basic knowledge of TWH is essential for learning about the culture from which the herbs originated. Mastering the qualities of each herb will support you in choosing similar herbs with indigenous roots or native to your area. In addition, TWH and curanderismo share many diagnostic methods and apothecary preparations, processes, and protocols.

CURANDERISMO AND ALLOPATHIC MEDICINE

Latine herbalism and curanderismo are practiced by many Latines in the USA—not just in the states with the highest populations of Mexican descendants (California, New Mexico, and Texas) but also in those with large Latine communities, such as New York, Florida, and Arizona. In some cases, herbs, rituals, and certain traditions have been passed down within families and are used in lieu of modern, or allopathic, medicine. As a result, medical doctors and hospitals often consult curanderas/os to better understand the healing culture of the community and offer services that align with their needs. This phenomenon is shared in detail from a curandera's point of view in *Woman Who Glows in the Dark* (2000) by Elena Avila and Joy Parker. In this popular book about curanderismo, Elena shares her story of empowerment as she transitioned from nurse to curandera to ultimately becoming a bridge between modern doctors and the Mexican-American community they served. Perhaps in the near future, there will be synergy between the services of curanderas/os and the modern medicine industry, much like there is with the services of a doula for the maternity industry.

NAVIGATING THIS BOOK

This book is not a scholarly or historical presentation. It is intended as a guide for readers to learn about all aspects of Latine herbalism and modern curanderismo. Let's recap what I have covered thus far:

- Definition of curanderismo
- Basics of the traditional school of curanderismo
- How curanderismo evolved as Latine herbalism
- The relationship between Traditional Western Herbalism and curanderismo, and the influence each has on the other

These topics lay the foundation that will be rounded out with basic anatomy (chapter 2), learning to make apothecary preparations (chapter 3), and herbal terminology (chapter 4), leading up to how to bring it all together with remedies and rituals.

Chapters 5–9 offer specifics; you will gain an understanding of what Latine herbalism and modern curanderismo offer for overcoming physical and energetic afflictions with positive results. These core chapters represent the five major energies that I believe reflect a balanced and complete being:

Sun Energy/*Energía del sol* (chapter 5) speaks to the digestive system. A well-functioning digestive system generates vitality in the body, hence an internal sun energy.

Moon Energy/*Energía de la luna* (chapter 6) covers how to regulate the nervous system. I relate the cool and soft energy of the moon to the energy we want to achieve from our nervous system when it is in balance.

Essence of the Breath/*Vibración del aliento* (chapter 7) is all about the breath. I share some tried-and-true recipes to keep the respiratory system open and clear.

Essence of the Heart/*Vibración del corazón* (chapter 8) covers the cardiovascular system while emphasizing the emotional heart.

Essence of the Flowers/*Espíritu de las flores* (chapter 9) shares my love of vibrational healing and how I approach and practice it as a modern curandera.

The last chapter will introduce you to modern curanderas/os, Latines who have strong personal practices in the healing arts and unique points of view. These practitioners may not call themselves curanderas/os but still use their gift/*don* to support others through life's challenges and ailments with grace and knowledge.

CHAPTER 2

ANATOMY BASICS

THE PHYSICAL BODY

Here, we will take an abbreviated look at the organ systems of the human body. During my first yoga certification, we learned about the yoga asanas (physical movements) in relation to the muscles, organs, and breath.

While this is not a medical text, it is important to introduce the organ systems for better clarity about the internal workings of the body. This understanding helps in choosing the appropriate apothecary preparation and in knowing how the herbs and botanicals function within the body or topical.

Integumentary System

The integumentary system is the outer layer of the body—the system we are typically most concerned with. Its purpose is to regulate body temperature, retain moisture, and absorb certain nutrients. It consists of hair, nails, skin, and sweat glands.

Muscular System

The muscular system is the most loved part of our bodies, aside from the outer skin. We talk about our muscles, shape them, and massage them. They are the reason our bodies defy gravity and stand upright. This system is made up of muscles, ligaments, and tendons.

Skeletal System

The skeletal system is our inner structure. It secures our muscles and houses most of our organs. In addition to their structural purpose, bones also store minerals and create blood cells in the bone marrow. This system consists of all bones—including the skull, spine, and rib cage—as well as joints and teeth.

Respiratory System

The respiratory system allows us to breathe. It takes oxygen into the lungs, transports it to the bloodstream, and releases carbon dioxide from the body. It includes the nose, mouth, throat, voice box, bronchi, and lungs.

Digestive System

The digestive system breaks down food to assimilate nutrients in the body and aids in the elimination of waste (urine and feces).

It includes the mouth, throat, esophagus, small intestine, large intestine, and rectum. The liver, gallbladder, and pancreas are accessory organs to this system.

Nervous System

The nervous system is the control system of the body. It sends messages from the brain to the muscles, organs, and glands and governs the parasympathetic and sympathetic systems. It consists of the brain, spinal cord, nerves (central nervous system and peripheral nervous system), and enteric nervous system.

Circulatory or Cardiovascular System

The cardiovascular system is responsible for blood circulation. In turn, the blood carries oxygen, nutrients, blood cells, and more throughout the body. This system includes the heart, blood vessels, and blood.

Reproductive System

The reproductive system is the only system that differs between the two sexes. Its function is to create offspring. It produces sperm (testicles), eggs (ovaries), menstrual blood (uterus), milk (mammary glands), and sex hormones. For women, it consists of the vagina, ovaries, uterus, fallopian tubes, and mammary glands. For men, it consists of the penis, testicles, scrotum, ductus deferens, and prostate gland.

Urinary System

The urinary system is responsible for eliminating liquid waste from the body, as well as balancing salts, electrolytes, and water in the blood. It includes the kidneys, bladder, urethra, and ureters.

Endocrine System

The endocrine system is a set of glands that release hormones to regulate a variety of bodily processes. Hormones are carried by the bloodstream and regulate the activity of cells. The endocrine system consists of the pineal gland, pituitary gland, thyroid gland, thymus, adrenal gland, pancreas, ovaries, and testicles.

Lymphatic System

The lymphatic system is a network of tissues and glands that carries lymph fluid—an infection-fighting fluid containing white blood cells that aids immunity—and helps remove waste from the bloodstream. It includes the thymus, lymphatic vessels, thoracic duct, spleen, lymph nodes, and red bone marrow.

The botanical remedios discussed in this book are intended to support the healing of the physical body. Previously, we introduced the main chapters. Four of them are dedicated to individual organ systems: the digestive system, the nervous system, the respiratory system, and the cardiovascular system.

THE VIBRATIONAL BODY

One system we don't often hear about is the vibrational body—also referred to as the energy body, the human energy field, the aura, or the spirit. Names shift depending on the modality and religious inclination used to describe it. It is called "prana" by the Indo-Asian, "chi" in Traditional Chinese Medicine (TCM), "mystery" by the American Indigenous, and "espíritu" by traditional curanderas/os. The idea of a vibrational body is becoming more mainstream, along with a consensus about the existence of an invisible, ethereal body that can influence the physical body. Some of the rituals shared in this book are rooted in this belief, which is why it's important to make a few observations.

Interaction with vibrational bodies requires perception. Because they do not manifest in a specific way or in a physical manner, awareness of them is subjective for each individual—people must be open to this belief and to their intuition. The concept of a vibrational body is not new—consider Reiki, sound healing, and the water studies by Masaru Emoto. Its foundational theory and concepts were also discussed by Barbara Ann Brennan in *Hands of Light* (1988). Brennan coined the term "human energy field," and her book provides ample detail about her personal experience in vibrational healing and how it manifested for her. Because it covers many facets of the vibrational body, I recommend this book for my Reiki and curanderismo students as a must-read even before our first meeting.

For those starting this journey who do not yet sense vibrational bodies or have not fine-tuned their perception, how do we know they are there without personal experience? In curanderismo, we examine emotions, thoughts, and mental afflictions for manifestations of vibrational energies that are out of alignment—specifically, the emotions of fear, anxiety, and worry. Curanderismo offers practices, and rituals, to bring these afflictions into alignment. In the coming chapters, I will share these with a modern approach. Vibrational healing, in particular, will be covered with more nuance in chapter 9, *Espíritu de las Flores*—Essence of the Flowers.

CHAPTER 3

APOTHECARY BASICS

THE HERBOLARIA TRADITION

In Mexico, Central America, and South America, along with parts of California and Texas, the word "*herbolaria*" refers to the school of botanicals (*L. materia medica*). It encompasses both the herbal preparations and the person (in the feminine) who administers the preparations—just as the word "apothecary" applies to both the store where medicines are sold and the person who sells them. These terms were commonly used until allopathic medicine became the medical standard. Today, "herbolaria" refers to the use of herbs and botanical preparations, and "apothecary" is interchangeable with the word "pharmacy" in the USA and parts of Europe. For our purposes in this book, I prefer "herbolaria" over "apothecary" because its root word, *hierba* (herb), honors the use of plants. According to Abigail

Aguilar Contreras, a professor at the UNAM Faculty of Sciences in Mexico City, "In pre-Hispanic times, plants were used for ailments and therapeutic practices"—hence, the word herbolaria, or an Indigenous-dialect form of the word, has been used for centuries within Mexico.

As mentioned in chapter 2, Latine herbalism and curanderismo are influenced by Traditional Western Herbalism principles; this is also true for herbolaria. We will learn about the use of *preparaciónes herbarias* (apothecary preparations) for easing afflictions. They have historically allowed for a more consistent use of botanicals across the seasons. For example, chamomile, used as a digestive in the summer, was commonly grown in people's gardens and was easily available. If you needed tea, it was right outside your door. But what happens in the winter, when snow covers the earth and no plants grow? The use of dried herbs or a premade tincture—a preparación—became the answer. In this chapter, we will learn about the different types of preparaciónes herbarias, as well as how to make them, and I will share both the Spanish and English terminologies.

HERBAL PREPARATIONS— *PREPARACIÓNES HERBARIAS*

Beyond bridging the seasons, preparaciónes herbarias are also made for ease of travel and consistency of use. When making the preparaciónes, there are two schools—one for those who make formulas by intuition, and one for those who use detailed recipes. Both approaches are valid, but note that if you want a truly consistent result with your preparaciónes, a recipe is best.

Once we have settled on which hierbas will be used, the preparación herbaria has three steps:

1. Choosing the botanicals' *structure*—root, leaf, or flower, and its *condition*—fresh or dried.
2. Deciding on the manner of application: topical or ingested.
3. Selecting the best *type* of preparación to use.

As a general rule, fresh botanicals are high in water content, while dried herbs are not. Fresh botanicals make for a lighter, fresher preparación. Dried botanicals tend to create a denser, concentrated formula. Fresh botanicals are best suited for poultices and extractions of water and alcohol. While dried botanicals can be used in all types of preparaciónes, it is important to note that fresh botanicals present a higher risk of developing mold and yeast, so a preservative to keep bacteria from growing is necessary. In curanderismo, the traditional preservative has been alcohol—such as *maíz* (wild corn or agua ardiente [high-proof sugarcane alcohol]). There are other options including brandy, wine, and jerez. *Jerez* (sherry) is a very popular traditional preservative used by curanderas/os in Mexico. Depending on the region, forms of high-proof Mezcal and Tequila are also used.

Most apothecary preparations are best packaged in glass bottles or jars, with amber-colored glass being the optimal choice. This hue minimizes sunlight exposure. Sunlight and heat deteriorate the efficacy of preparaciónes and speed up the evaporation process, spoiling the end result. Be sure to label all packaging before storing, with as much information as possible—including common name, Indigenous name, and Latin name (Latin names are used today to cross reference with other herbalists in other countries when sharing information), date made, date of expiration, description and indications, full ingredients, and dose. If you gather or forage for your own hierbas, it is also advisable to include the place and season on the label.

Although the process of making preparaciónes herbarias might seem straightforward, in curanderismo, we also consider the don of the maker along with the therapeutic value of the botanicals, as well as the vibration and energy of the time and space. Many curanderas/os will choose auspicious times, such as a festive full moon or seasonal equinox, to enhance the remedios. They might also offer prayers and incantations to enhance the energetic benefits. When making your preparaciónes herbarias, do so with JOY! Be "in-spirited" to collaborate with Nature in sharing her bounty of well-being with yourself and those around you.

UTENSILS—*EQUIPO*

Certain accessories will help make the creation of your remedios easy and fun. Following is a list of what you will need. Making preparaciónes herbarias is similar to cooking; the utensils and supplies are similar, but it is a good idea to keep them separate, as some hierbas can stain or leave behind small traces that could contaminate your food. I recommend using either glass or stainless steel; these materials are referred to as nonporous in the food industry, as they do not absorb oils, scents, or particles and are easy to clean and sterilize.

Cotton muslin or cheesecloth—In some cases, you'll want to use fabrics made of cotton, such as cheesecloth or muslin, for straining. These are usually used once and then composted. Alternatively, you can use a superfine metal strainer.

Double boiler—Many recipes call for indirect heat, and double boilers present the safest method for that purpose. The size depends on how much you plan to make; you can start with a small double boiler and graduate to a larger one. There are many types of double boilers, but the one *you* prefer is the one that works best. I have a glass one that a friend gifted me for my birthday, and I treasure it! If a double boiler is not available, you can use a small pot over a larger pot, ensuring that it sits within the opening but does not touch the bottom. If you choose this method, the top pot should be made of glass, stainless steel, or coated ceramic. Never use nonstick, cast iron, or aluminum for your top pot, as these materials can react with some of the bases and hierbas and spoil your preparaciónes.

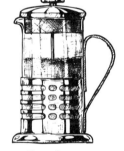

French press—Used for ease of straining when making large amounts of infusions or extractions. While not always necessary, it is simple and easy to use.

Funnel—A funnel makes for easy transfer from larger to smaller containers. When possible, stainless steel is preferred.

French press

General utensils—While wooden utensils may create a pretty mental picture, stainless steel is preferred. Wood absorbs particles and scents. If used for heating wax, for example, it can be difficult to clean. Stainless steel utensils are lightweight and easy to maintain. I recommend having a variety of sizes, as it's better to have extra than not enough.

Glass jars—Glass jars, usually mason jars, are used for storing raw materials and final preparaciónes. Having various sizes is always helpful. Unless otherwise stated, "mason jar" in this book refers to the standard 1-quart size with a metal lid.

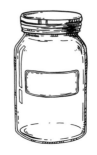

Glass or metal packaging—Once we are ready to use the preparaciónes, we can transfer them from our storage or herbolaria to final packaging. Begin with mason jars and "Boston" round bottles, glass dropper bottles, small metal tins, and glass mist bottles.

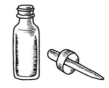

Mason jar (top) and Boston round bottle

Heat source—For most of us, the kitchen is where the major heat source, or stove, is located and where we will create our formulas. However, some may want to establish a separate space and install a portable heat source. Either method works well; just be sure never to leave it unattended and to turn it off completely when finished.

Hot-water kettle—Although electrical kettles are popular, I still prefer the stovetop version, as well as the old-fashioned method of using a pot to boil water.

Measuring cups—Traditional glass cups work very well; they are durable and easy to

Hot-water kettle

use. The first ones I bought, which I still use, were from a thrift store. Because they are glass, sterilizing them is easy, and I don't worry about contamination. As with any of the other utensils, avoid plastic, as it is porous and will leave behind microplastic particles over time, which we don't want in our preparaciónes.

Mortar and pestle/blender—For grinding and mixing materials, the blender has largely replaced the mortar and pestle. I seldom use a mortar and pestle, as it requires not only time but skill to achieve a good blend. My father, however, preferred using a mortar and pestle for his preparaciónes, which were always with fresh hierbas, and the metal of the blender would oxidize them.

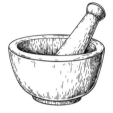
Mortar and pestle

Pots—Glass, stainless steel, or coated ceramic are good choices.

Scale—A scale is essential for those of us in the "detailed recipe" school; it is also important when creating new recipes or ones we might want to replicate.

Strainer—Stainless steel strainers are recommended, as they are nonporous and easy to clean and sterilize.

Thermometer—Both infrared and digital thermometers work well.

Wooden craft sticks—Although stainless steel works best in most cases, wooden craft sticks are the exception, especially for making wax-blended preparaciónes. Since it is difficult to clean wax, and you don't want to clog your pipes, I suggest using wooden sticks for scraping instead of utensils, and then composting them. They go right back to the Earth. If you don't have compost or a place to bury the sticks, cleaning wax involves a three-step process. First, clean the utensils and pots with paper while still warm and the wax is liquid; I use newspaper. Second, wash with hot, soapy water. Third, dry and wipe with alcohol to eliminate any residue.

MATERIALS— *MATERIA PRIMA*

Preparaciónes herbarias are made from *materia prima* (raw materials). These include oils, alcohols, and botanicals in their raw states. The basic materials you will need are:

Alcohol—Within Latine herbalism and curanderismo, *aguardiente* (sugarcane alcohol—literally, "stinging water") is most prevalent. In Mexico, it is sometimes called *alcohol destilado* (distilled alcohol) to differentiate it from synthetic alcohols such as denatured alcohol and isopropyl alcohol. The choice of alcohol for the final preparaciónes will be based on the properties of the alcohol and, if ingested, its flavor. Other choices include alcohol de maíz, vodka, jerez, brandy, and wine.

Botanicals—Botanicals, or hierbas, are at the core of formulating a preparación. Which hierba to use depends on the ailment; the formula will dictate how to use it. Frequency and length of treatment depend on the ailment and ultimately on the curandera/o or Latine herbalist's suggestion.

Carrier oils—These are oils that "carry" the therapeutic properties of the botanicals. I favor grapeseed oil because it is fast-absorbing and nongreasy. Other oils include coconut oil, olive oil, sunflower oil, and sweet almond oil. You will discover which oils' properties work best in your formulas through trial and error.

Essential oils—These are concentrated distillations of fresh botanicals. Only minute amounts are needed to produce strong formulas. Historically, essential oils were made for their scents; it was believed that they carried the same properties as the physical hierbas. Hence the name represented the "essence" of the plant. While essential oils are still popular today, in curanderismo and Latine herbalism, we predominantly work with botanicals in their original, raw form. If you feel called to use essential oils, educate yourself on best practices and never ingest them.

Water—Water is used for the leading type of preparación—water infusions, also known as herbal tea. Because the resulting preparación is for ingestion, the water used should be of the highest quality available; natural or spring water is preferred—but definitely not tap water or even filtered water. If spring water is unavailable, purified water is a good substitute.

Waxes—Beeswax is traditionally used in formulating preparaciónes, but with the rise of veganism, plant-based waxes such as *candelilla* (Mexican plant wax) and *carnauba* (Brazilian palm wax), derived from flowers and leaves, have become more available. Sourcing waxes from sustainable farms with organic practices is ideal.

SPACE—
SITIO DE CREACIÓN

Along with your supplies and materials, the physical space where you will create your preparaciónes herbarias is important. It should be clean and orderly. Many will use the kitchen as this space; make sure it is clean and sanitized before and after you use it. Keep the supplies organized and separate from kitchen utensils. Your materials should be stored in a cool, dry place away from direct sunlight. These best practices will support the making of preparaciónes that are safe, clean, and accurate.

While making your preparaciónes, the accompaniment of devotional music, songs, or mantras is highly recommended, as these will enhance your formulas vibrationally and energetically. All liquids, especially water, have the capacity to hold energy in their molecular structure, as demonstrated by Dr. Emoto's water experiments in his book, *The Hidden Messages in Water* (Atria, 2005). Using chanting, prayer, song, or music will infuse your preparations with positive energies.

TYPES OF PREPARACIÓNES HERBARIAS

Poultice—*Cataplasma o fomento natural*

A poultice is the direct application of an herbal mixture on the skin. Traditionally, the fresh herb is made into a paste using a mortar and pestle. This method is still practiced in many pueblos and by many curanderas/os. Some Indigenous tribes also chew the fresh herbs, benefiting from the therapeutics of the hierbas in two forms, ingested and topically. My father used fomentos for all his physical pains. I watched him many times process the *hierbitas* by hand and add his magic touch to the paste. Sometimes, he would do this for others and lovingly wrap the fresh paste for delivery.

Basic Preparation: Gather or measure out enough fresh plant material to cover the affected area of skin. Using a blender on low speed or a mortar and pestle, macerate the hierbas until a wet paste results. Adding a water infusion or infused oil can enhance the moistness, if necessary. Apply the paste to the skin and cover with waterproof material; traditionally a plastic bag is used but today there are many options like reusable beeswax wraps and compostable wraps or bags.

When to Use: For topical ailments that require immediate attention.

General Shelf Life: 1 use.

Fomentation—*Fomento de tela*

Fomentation is a gentler form of poultice, using a cloth to apply liquid extractions or infused oil to the skin. This method can be used with children and the elderly. Warming the oils or extractions can increase the therapeutic benefits. Traditionally, cotton fabric with a high thread count is used. Flannel or soft brushed cotton also work well.

Basic Preparation: Saturate the fabric with liquid and apply it to the affected area. Wrap it with waterproof material.

When to Use: Fomentation can be used for physical ailments of a long-term nature.

General Shelf Life: 1 use for water extractions; 2–3 uses for oil-infused fomentations.

Infusions—*Infusiones*

Water Infusion—*Infusión de hierbas o tisana*

The original water infusion is the age-old therapeutic tea. The difference between a "tea" and a "therapeutic tea" lies in the steep time and the manner in which it is administered. For water infusions, hierbas are most efficiently brewed in a French press. The extended steep time draws out the herb properties and produces a concentrated infusion. It can be taken as is or diluted further, depending on the suggested dose. The taste is often strong enough to warrant the addition of honey or another sweetener. Either fresh or dried hierbas can be used. Note that it is becoming more common among tea lovers and herbalists to use the word "tea" to represent water infusions of only the plant *Camellia sinesis* and calling all other plant infusions *tisanes.*

Basic Preparation: Use 2 tablespoons of hierbas per 1 cup of water. Add hot water (just boiled) to the hierbas, cover, and steep for 4–8 hours. I learned from both family lineage and studies with other curanderas/os that fresh flowers, seeds, leaves, stems, and roots should be steeped for 4–5 hours; dried flowers and some seeds for 4 hours; and dried leaves, stems, and some roots for 6–8 hours. Most dried roots require 8 hours to steep, or a decoction method is used. The tea is strained and served at room temperature or heated. To alter its flavor, tea can be sweetened and/or diluted.

When to Use: Water infusions (therapeutic teas) are taken orally for ailments of a long-term nature. Consistent use will help improve, support, and restore well-being.

General Shelf Life: One to two days at room temperature or three to four days in the refrigerator.

Decoction—*Decocción*

A decoction is a water infusion usually reserved for hard-to-extract materials such as roots and some medicinal mushrooms. They are sometimes mixed with alcohol for long-term storage.

Basic Preparation: Use 2–4 tablespoons of hierba per 1 cup of water. Bring the water to a boil, add the hierbas, and reduce to a simmer, uncovered, until ¼ of the water has evaporated. Cool; serve at room temperature. This is the original form of syrup and can be sweetened to taste.

When to Use: Decoctions can replace therapeutic teas (water infusions) for long-term ailments.

General Shelf Life: After cooling, decoctions can be stored one to two days at room temperature or three to four days refrigerated.

Oil Infusion—*Infusión de aceite o aceite infusionado*

In an oil infusion, the therapeutic properties of hierbas are infused into a carrier oil. The traditional method is solar infusion, where the vessel containing the formula is heated by the sun for a full lunar cycle, or approximately thirty days. Dried herbs are preferred for this method, as oil and water do not mix, and the excess moisture in fresh herbs can ruin the preparation. The nontraditional, much quicker method is a slow-heat infusion over a stovetop.

Basic Preparation: Use a 1:2 ratio of hierba to oil. Add all ingredients to a jar, cover with a tight lid, and place it where it will receive sunlight for 8–12 hours a day. Shake two to three times a week for one lunar cycle. The stovetop method requires the same herb-to-oil ratio but is heated over a slow simmer in a double boiler for 3–6 hours. It can also be made in a slow cooker at a low temperature, infusing for 2–4 hours.

When to Use: Oil infusions are primarily used topically; they are rarely taken orally except for culinary oils. In either instance, they are used for short-term ailments. Oil infusions are also used in making "compound" or combination preparaciónes herbarias, in which two preparations are combined to make one. Balms and creams are made in this fashion.

General Shelf Life: Up to one year for infused oils made with dried materials; two to six weeks if fresh materials are used.

Extractions—*Extracciones*

Cold Water Extractions—*Aguas frescas*

Aguas frescas (fresh waters) are extractions of fresh hierbas in water at room temperature. This particular method is employed in the smaller pueblos in Mexico as part of the local *gastronomía* (gastronomy). It is also used as a preventative measure when allopathic care is not within reach. Aguas frescas are made by blending water with fresh hierbas, fruit, flowers, nuts, or seeds. A favorite agua fresca of mine is alfalfa and lemon; it has a crisp, green flavor that is unique! I believe this is a simpler way to juice fruits and vegetables, with equivalent therapeutic properties to juicing.

Basic Preparation: Use a 1:2 ratio of hierba to water. Blend at high speed until completely mixed; strain out all pulp; serve chilled, with or without ice.

When to Use: Ingested as a digestive with food or for a short-term ailment.

General Shelf Life: Not stored; ingest immediately.

Tinctures—*Tinturas*

Tinctures are traditionally made with an alcohol base. Traditional Western Herbalism practices use 60- to 80-proof alcohol, usually vodka, as the customary choice. In the USA, the use of "moonshine" and other high-content artisanal alcohols has become popular. In Mexico, as well as Central and South America, brandy, sherry, and wine are commonly used. In my experience, tinctures made with brandy and wine make a sweeter formula. The use of alcohol is twofold: to extract constituents (water) and to preserve (alcohol) the preparación. Tinctures are more concentrated than therapeutic teas (water infusions) and in general are more convenient to use. They have a longer shelf life because they can be made in one batch and preserved, instead of making a new serving for each use. Tinctures take approximately a full lunar cycle to extract the herbal constituents, unless you choose the decoction method. Both fresh and dried hierbas are suitable for this type of preparación and can yield distinctly different flavors and aromas. More about the use of fresh versus dried botanicals is found in the individual chapters.

Basic Preparation: Use a 1:2 ratio of botanicals to alcohol. Add all ingredients to a jar and place it away from sunlight in a cool area for a full lunar cycle, shaking every other day. When ready, pour into dropper bottles for easy dosing and store in a cool, shaded area.

When to Use: Tinctures can replace therapeutic teas (water infusions) for ease of use. If the alcohol taste is strong, add the tincture to warm water to evaporate the alcohol. Although traditionally made to be ingested, some tinctures can be used topically.

General Shelf Life: One to two years.

Glycerin Tinctures—*Tinturas de glicerina*

Glycerin tinctures are used when alcohol is not recommended. They are a sweet and softer extraction, particularly used for children and when honey is not suitable. *Note:* Take care to use a plant-based glycerin, as animal- and petroleum-based versions also exist. Unlike other water-extraction bases, glycerin can also serve as a simple preservative, although with a shorter shelf life than alcohol tinctures.

Basic Preparation:. Part one: calculate the total glycerine tincture. (Example: 32 ounces.) Part two: Calculate 3 parts glycerine to 1 part water. (Example: 24 ounces of glycerine, 8 ounces of water.) Part three: Prepare 1 part botanical to 2 parts of the water total. (Example: 4 ounces botanicals, 8 ounces water.) Bring the water to a boil, rest for a minute, and add the botanicals. Let steep for 30 minutes. Combine with the glycerin and mix well. Store in a cool, shaded area away from sunlight for a full lunar cycle. Shake three times a week; you'll notice the formula getting deeper in color. When ready, strain fully and store in large containers until ready to dispense into smaller bottles.

When to Use: As a replacement for alcohol tinctures for short- and long-term ailments.

General Shelf Life: One year.

Infused Vinegar—*Infusión de vinagre o vinagre aromatizado*

If you are concerned about alcohol consumption, vinegar can be used to replace the alcohol in the same preparation as a tincture, described previously. However, some botanicals react poorly to vinegar and do not tincture well, leaving behind a smelly residue that eventually turns sour and ruins the final preparation. I encourage making a microbatch to test things out before attempting a large batch. It is also important to note that vinegar reacts with metal. Avoid using metal for mixing, storing, and even serving (this includes spoons, containers, and lids). Fresh or dried hierbas can be used; however, using fresh hierbas will shorten the process and life of this tincture.

Basic Preparation: Use a 1:2 ratio of botanicals to vinegar. Add all of the ingredients to a jar, close with a plastic lid, and place away from sunlight in a cool area for half a moon cycle (approximately fifteen days, or seven to ten days if using fresh hierbas), mixing every other day. If the strength is not as desired, allow another fifteen days of extraction. Strain well; sometimes I double strain. Store in large glass containers with plastic lids until ready to use and dispense into smaller bottles for dosing. Always shake infused vinegars before decanting (opening) the storage bottle. Sediment is prominent in infused vinegars, especially when using vinegars with a vinegar mother.

When to Use: Infused vinegars are used for short-term ailments, especially of a respiratory nature, as the vinegar supports the opening of the lungs and eases breathing.

General Shelf Life: When made with dried materials: one year. When made with fresh materials: two to three weeks, check before use.

Essential Oils—*Aceites esenciales*

Essential oils are volatile alcohols extracted through distillation, expression, or extraction from plant material. They are highly concentrated and must be diluted before use. Originally, essential oils were a byproduct of the distillation process. As their name implies, they were considered the "essence" of the hierba and were highly valued. In the pursuit of natural scents, essential oils have largely replaced fragrance oils. However, we have no evidence that this use is safe long-term. Today, essential oils are overused in cosmetics, flavors, and bath products. I suggest they be used minimally and, due to their concentration, only topically and highly diluted. I will not cover the distillation, expression, or extraction methods, as that would require an entire book, but I include the dilution method suggested by aromatherapists for wellness support. Store all essential oils away from sunlight and heat; never use them undiluted, and never take them orally.

Basic Preparation: Sold at wellness or specialty stores. The recommended dilution rate is 4–8 drops of essential oil per 1 ounce (by weight) of carrier oil.

When to Use: Often used along with compound preparations. Recommended for topical use only and short-term relief.

General Shelf Life: One year.

Aromatic Waters—*Aguas florales o aguas aromáticas de (nombre de la hierba) o aguas distiladas de (nombre de la hierba) o agua de (nombre de la hierba)*

Aromatic waters are also called hydrosols. They contain the same volatile alcohols as essential oils but at much lower concentrations. Traditionally, the distillation process for extracting the essence from hierbas resulted in *agua aromática*, with essential oils as the byproduct. They tended to be quite stable and possessed a long shelf life. Today, most aromatic waters contain preservatives and are not to be used for ingestion. Curanderas/os continue to use aromatic waters, for topical purposes, especially for rituals and limpias.

Basic Preparation: Sold at wellness or specialty stores. Transfer to a glass container if the original package is plastic, and store in a cool, dry place away from sunlight. Pour into mist bottles for use.

When to Use: Use topically for short- and long-term ailments.

General Shelf Life: One year.

Compounds—*Compuestos*

Compounds occur when two or more ingredients are combined to make one preparation. Traditional compounds include balms; others are invented on the spot, such as mixing a glycerin tincture with a water infusion, resulting in a new preparation.

Balm/Salve/Ointment—*Crema/pomada/ungüento*

With a thicker consistency than liquids, balms, salves, and ointments are fundamentally the same and are used for applying the therapeutic properties of hierbas to the skin. They are also convenient to travel with and have better shelf lives than infused oils. Although their consistency may vary, all three are commonly called *ungüentos*, even when it is a balm or a salve. They are traditionally a combination of oil and wax, sometimes with added essential oils, powders, or other plant material. Curanderas/os—particularly hueseras/os and parteras/os—are well known for their custom ungüentos for supporting physical healing.

In preparing compounds, it is important to understand the alchemical quality of heat as a binder. The longer the wax and oil can merge while heated, the more uniform the final product will be, regardless of its thickness. Compounds take time and cannot be rushed. I suggest not beginning your journey of preparaciónes herbarias with a balm or salve; start with an infusion and slowly work up to compounds.

Balms—*Crema o bálsamo:* Balms have a thick, hard consistency that contains more wax than other compounds. They are a good choice for hot climates and for use during the summer months. Balms are usually massaged into the skin, and the massage itself is also a form of healing, especially from a huesera/o or partera/o.

Ratio: 1 cup oil to 1.5 ounces wax (weight).

Salves—*Pomada:* Salves have a medium consistency, and when pressed, their density easily breaks down. They are easily applied to the skin, sometimes leaving a bit of wax on the surface. Salves are commonly found commercially, more so than balms or ointments; the terms "balm" and "salve" are often used interchangeably.

Ratio: 1 cup oil to 1 ounce wax (weight).

Ointments—*Ungüento:* Ointments can resemble lotions. With a higher oil content, they are easily spread and applied to the skin, typically without rubbing it in. Ointments rest on the upper dermis and are covered with gauze or cloth to allow them to work their magic. Due to their high oil content, ointments will melt at high temperatures.

Ratio: 1 cup oil to 0.75 ounce wax (weight).

Basic Preparation for Balms, Salves, and Ointments: In a double boiler, heat the wax until it is fully melted. Add the oil. The wax will harden temporarily, but allow it to melt again. Heat for 10–15 minutes, mixing slowly on occasion. Remove it from the heat, mix, and cool for 5 minutes. Add any additives. Pour into individual containers for storage. Let cool completely before use. As you become more acquainted with making these, you might want to monitor the temperature to ensure consistent preparaciónes.

When to Use: Used topically for short-term ailments.

General Shelf Life: Balms: one to two years; salves and ointments: one year.

Elixirs—*Tónicos o jarabes*

Tónicos are considered a "poor man's tincture"; their use is very common in curanderismo. Sometimes called syrups, elixirs are a combination of water extractions and alcohols. They can preserve therapeutic teas (water infusions) for a long shelf life, or they can be diluted further with water or juice and served; sometimes, they are merely watered-down tinctures. Because you control the water-to-alcohol ratio, elixirs can be customized—it all depends on the curandera/o, proving again that curanderismo is a living tradition with diversity. Elixirs are traditionally consumed at once, but if they are to be stored, use glass containers and keep them in a cool area away from sunlight. Transfer to glass bottles for administering.

Basic Preparation: Mix 3 parts tea/decoction to 1 part alcohol of your choice.

When to Use: Elixirs are used for quick consumption for short-term ailments or as a preventative remedio.

General Shelf Life: Two weeks to one year, depending on the water ratio; the more water, the shorter the shelf life.

BUILDING A HOME HERBOLARIA

Aside from being a place to house your supplies and materials and to make preparaciónes, a home herbolaria is a way to stay connected to Nature. You may have noticed that curanderismo and Latine herbalism represent an extension of the use of the elements for personal self-discovery and wellness. A home herbolaria will facilitate the use of hierbas and remedios by keeping them all at your fingertips.

The organization of the herbs in a home herbolaria ultimately depends on the person: how you use your hierbas and what your priorities are. I tend to organize my herbolaria with the most used items in the front, on easy-to-reach shelves, and the least used items in the back rows or on the top and bottom shelves. I also like to rotate the hierbas by season. Cooling hierbas are up front in the summer, switching out to warming hierbas in the winter. Find what works for you, and your herbolaria will be a place where you can house preparaciónes for remedios y rituales to share with all.

Storage of your utensils, raw materials, and finished products is key. I have two large shelving units with doors in proximity to the kitchen. One unit holds packaging, essential oils, carrier oils, butters, waxes, and finished preparaciónes. The other holds dried herbs, tinctures, infused vinegars, and two shelves of specialized tea-ware and Chinese teas, as I also practice Cha Dao—a meditative tea ceremony. My utensils are stored in a separate, smaller shelving unit. Although many keep the herbolaria on kitchen shelves and may not have space to do otherwise, I recommend keeping the hierbas and raw materials protected behind doors, as I find this helps keep the physical and vibrational energies more stable.

CHAPTER 4

HERBAL TERMINOLOGY

Let's explore the way plants grow and the parts of plants used in curanderismo and Latine herbalism. This will round out the basics—along with information about the energetics of plants, anatomical systems, and preparaciónes herbarias—before we begin to explore the remedios y rituales. Perhaps now is a good time to brew a simple cup of tea before reading about what exactly might be in your cup.

If you already grow your own herbs, some of this may be redundant; but if you do not, Chart C on page 48 presents a simplified growth cycle of plants. I encourage you to begin the quest of at least planting one seed and watching it grow into a full plant, perhaps allowing it to flower and fruit; this will connect you more deeply to the natural world.

Chart C: Growth Cycle Graph

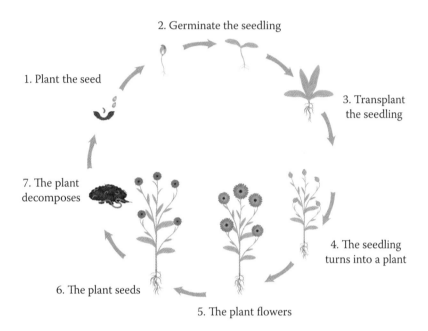

2. Germinate the seedling

1. Plant the seed

3. Transplant the seedling

7. The plant decomposes

4. The seedling turns into a plant

6. The plant seeds

5. The plant flowers

In the growth process, four points of harvest occur: the plant stage, in which leaves and stems are harvested; the flower stage; the fruit stage; and the root stage at the end of the plant's life, just before decomposition. It is important to understand the cycle of plants to harvest each part at the height of its vitality. For example, if you grow chamomile, you would want to wait until the flowering stage to harvest the plant for optimal therapeutic benefit.

It is also important to familiarize yourself with the plant parts. Chart D presents a drawing of the *romero* (rosemary) herb to better understand a plant's anatomy.

Chart D: Rosemary Drawing

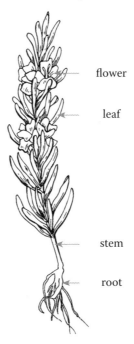

flower

leaf

stem

root

In the coming chapters, we will see how different parts of the plant hold different therapeutic benefits. While some are valued for their flowers and others for their roots, many hierbas hold value in all their parts, and knowing when to use each is important. Now that you have a bit more knowledge of the basics, let us delve into the details about when and how to use plants.

CHAPTER 5

ENERGÍA DEL SOL—
SUN ENERGY

In Mexico, a prevailing belief holds that the womb, the place of physical creation, mirrors the place of creativity in the vibrational body. Moreover, the belly button is the source of power and connection to the vibrational body, as it serves as the connection and lifeline—the umbilical cord—to our mothers. This is why many traditional curanderas/os wear a red belt when performing rituals. It is seen as a form of protection for their vibrational body and a way to contain and protect energy while performing rituals in the liminal, vibrational spaces.

The belly button area is equally important in Ayurveda and yogic philosophy. Ayurvedic philosophy mentions an inner fire, which relates to the digestive fire, or Agni, as it is called in Ayurveda. When Agni is out of balance, the physical body is similarly unbalanced, and harmony is out of reach. For this reason, food is considered a form of medicine, as how you eat, when you eat, and what you eat will affect your physical body. In yogic "subtle body" philosophy, the Manipura chakra, or third chakra, is located in the belly. It is believed that this chakra holds the element of fire as well as the seat of vibrational power and confidence. As an element, fire has a transformative quality; whatever passes through fire transforms into something different from its original form. An example is water; when water is heated, it becomes steam. So it is with Agni at the Manipura chakra; it is the place of transformation in the physical and vibrational body, where food turns into body fuel and the breath builds vitality.

It is interesting to see how different cultures hold the center of the body as a place of power and transformation. I have found in my personal experience working with clients and students of curanderismo and yoga philosophy that the belly button area can hold the power of confidence, the power of digestion, the power of motivation, and the power to transform when that elemental essence is summoned. For this reason, I see a metaphorical sun at the site of the belly: the sun holds elemental qualities of fire as well as transformative power within Nature.

As the sun and fire can transform, so can the digestive system. The food and water we ingest transform into the energy and nutrients we need to survive daily. When our digestive system is off, not only do we become weak and sickly, but external viruses can also take hold of our bodies. How we feed our bodies is so important! This is why the remedios in this chapter are specific to certain ailments and also provide preventative measures to support overall wellness. This chapter, along with the next three, will be divided into two sections: remedios (remedies) and rituales (rituals). You will find recipes in each section with specific herbs to ease both the physical and vibrational bodies.

REMEDIES—*REMEDIOS*

Some of the best digestive remedios are simple, and many of the herbs used in curanderismo are likely already familiar to you. As the herbs are introduced, you will begin to see and understand the underlying qualities of Traditional Western Herbalism presented in chapter 1. Generally, digestive issues are considered ailments resulting from too much heat and air in the digestive system. Indigestion and intestinal discomfort are typical maladies. The remedios offered here are predominantly of a cooling and drying quality.

Mint Tea ❀ *Te de yerba buena*

Peppermint (*L. Mentha x piperita*)—*Yerba buena*

ENERGY: Cold/dry | **TASTE:** Bitter | **PLANT PART USED:** Leaf and stem

This tea is served at the first sign of indigestion or gas. When someone overeats or eats food that is not well digested, all Mexican mothers, aunts, and grandmothers make a strong cup of *té de yerba buena* (mint tea). This tea is made by boiling the fresh mint hierba and adding a heaping spoonful of sugar. Drink quickly. *Yerba buena* (literally, "good herb") includes many mint herbs and varies by region; it can refer to spearmint, peppermint, or any of the mint family varieties. The aromatic and

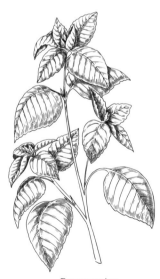

Peppermint

bitter taste of all mints works well for this tea. If you cannot grow it yourself, all Latine food markets carry fresh bunches in the produce sections. If you want to always be prepared, store dried peppermint herb in your herbolaria as a perfect substitute for yerba buena. The preparation of fresh hierba tea differs from the therapeutic tea (Water Infusion, page 34) and is a lighter decoction.

Mint Tea with Fresh Herbs Recipe

YIELD: approximately 2 cups

> ½ cup mint leaves
> 2 cups water
> preferred sweetener

> Bring the water to a boil, add the mint leaves, and simmer for up to 10 minutes. Remove from heat and let it rest for a minute; strain and serve. Add sweetener to taste.

Suggested Use: Drink immediately, 1 cup every 2 hours.

Mint Tea with Dried Herbs Recipe

YIELD: approximately 2 cups

> 1 tablespoon dried peppermint hierba
> 2 cups water
> preferred sweetener

> Bring the water to a boil, add the peppermint hierba, and remove from heat. Steep for 1 hour. Strain; reheat before serving. Add sweetener to taste.

Suggested Use: Drink immediately, 1 cup every 2 hours.

Hibiscus Tea ✿ *Agua de jamaica*

Hibiscus (*L. Hibiscus sabdariffa*)—*Flor de jamaica*

ENERGY: Cold/dry | **TASTE:** Bitter | **PLANT PART USED:** Flower bud or calyx.

There is a misconception that this tea is made with the bloomed flower, but in fact, it is made with the bud before flowering. If you harvest it fresh, take care to remove the seeds before using or drying.

There is not a *taquería* (taco stand) in Mexico that doesn't serve iced *agua de Jamaica* (hibiscus tea). This tea helps ease digestion as a preventative drink and is usually made to be served cold, but when té de yerba buena is unavailable for hot tea, hibiscus is an excellent alternative. Agua de Jamaica is a rich, concentrated liquid; it is one of my favorite *aguas* (teas). My godmother Esther makes this at her restaurant, and it is by far the most popular drink. I am sharing a smaller version of her recipe, as she makes over 10 gallons a day! When making agua de Jamaica, dried hierba is preferred. Here is a tip when making large batches of teas and decoctions: they can be frozen for later use.

Hibiscus Tea Recipe

YIELD: approximately 5 cups of concentrate

2 cups whole dried hibiscus flowers

6 cups water, room temperature

muslin sieve

preferred sweetener

Mix the hibiscus flowers and water in a large pot, cover, and steep overnight. The next morning, bring it to a boil, remove from heat, and steep until it reaches room temperature again. Strain through a muslin sieve, squeezing as you strain to extract all the herbal goodness. The concentrate can be frozen in ice cube trays or refrigerated for dilution at the time of serving. To dilute, use 1 part concentrate to 1 part water. Add sweetener to taste when served, or drink tart if you prefer; serve over ice.

Suggested Use: Serve with meals; drink 8–10 ounces as a preventative for indigestion and bloating.

Digestive Lemonade ✿ *Limonada Cubana*

Lemon (*L. Citrus limon*)—*Limón*

ENERGY: Lemon—cold/dry; baking soda is alkaline = neutral | **TASTE:** Bitter | **PLANT PART USED:** Fresh juice

My father taught me this digestive *remedio*. He would mix this *limonada* when I had an upset stomach with loose bowels. It also works for digestive support after overeating or ingesting fatty foods and as heartburn relief. This is one of those *remedios* that can be used anywhere you find lemons or limes and baking soda. It has supported me more than once in my many travels. While not many people know this recipe in Mexico, many Cuban families I know have made the bubbly brew when called for at gatherings. I think of this as the original effervescent, alkalizing

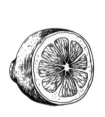
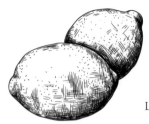

Lemons

antacid. The acidity of the lemon and the alkalizing pH of baking soda work together to relieve the extremes that cause indigestion.

Digestive Lemonade Recipe

YIELD: approximately 1 cup

juice of half a lemon

4–6 ounces water, cool or room temperature

½ tablespoon baking soda

preferred sweetener

Add the lemon juice, water, and sweetener to a glass; mix well to dissolve the sweetener. Add the baking soda and watch the mixture bubble up! Drink quickly; if there is sediment, add more water to ingest it all. If you prefer, the sweetener can be avoided.

Suggested Use: Make and drink immediately at the first sign of heartburn, flatulence, or loose bowels.

NOURISHING FOODS

As a preventative method, nourishing foods are essential to keep the digestive system flowing. Raising the sun energy of the digestive system requires eating foods that are simple to digest. I share two nourishing recipes here that are easy to make. I often recommend these recipes to my clients to cleanse the digestive system and when a mono diet can be useful.

In the tradition of curanderismo, laxatives are often seen as necessary when digestive issues arise, but I prefer a gentler cleanse to reset the digestive fire.

Chicken Broth ✿ *Caldo de gallina*

While beef broth has long been popular among the wellness crowd for its nutritious value, in Mexico, chicken broth has been used since pre-Hispanic times to fortify children, elders, and the sickly. You can often find this broth as a staple on menus at many *fondas* (artisanal cafes) in the pueblos. Unlike beef broth, caldo de gallina is made with the entire chicken; but as the Spanish name implies, a *gallina* (female hen), usually older, is specifically preferred. The broth is a gelatinous, nutrient-dense liquid that is said metaphorically to hold the power to *revivir un muerto* (revive the dead). It is also used as a hangover and flu remedio. This is my own recipe, modified to serve as a mono diet for a week.

Chicken Broth Recipe

YIELD: approximately 1½ gallons of broth

2 tablespoons avocado oil

1 cup diced onions

1 cup diced carrots

1 cup diced celery

¼ cup chopped garlic

1 hen or chicken (approximately 2½ pounds)

2 gallons distilled water

2 tablespoons apple cider vinegar

handful fresh parsley, washed and uncut

cooked rice (optional)

diced broccoli (optional)

shredded carrots (optional)

Ask your butcher to cut the hen into quarters and to cut across the drumsticks to expose the bone marrow. Retain the innards and neck. In a large pot, add the avocado oil and sauté the onions until tender. Add the carrots, celery, and garlic and sauté for another 5 minutes.

Add the hen pieces, skin side down, and brown lightly for about 8 minutes. Turn the pieces over and cook another 8 minutes. Slowly add 1 cup of water to deglaze, scraping any stuck meat or vegetables from the bottom of the pan. Add the remaining water and bring to a boil. Reduce the heat and simmer for 3 hours, lightly covered, mixing once or twice an hour. Remove from heat and add the apple cider vinegar, mixing slowly. Add the parsley to the top of the pot without mixing it in and let cool for an hour. Remove the hen pieces and parsley. If the broth is gelatinous, heat it until it liquefies, but avoid boiling. Strain the remaining vegetables from the broth. You will have two functional items from this recipe: the strained broth without vegetable, and the chicken meat. Both can be frozen until ready to use. I freeze them in portions of two servings for easy defrosting.

Suggested Serving:

- *As a cleanse:* Reheat the broth and serve with cooked rice and raw vegetables. I suggest a three-day cleanse using this broth to reset the digestive system.

- *For nourishment:* Reheat the broth and add shredded hen meat, vegetables, and cooked potatoes for a more filling soup version.

- *Optional:* Add medicinal mushrooms at the simmer stage to raise the herbal potency of this incredible dish. Medicinal mushrooms grow on wood, not in the earth; they include reishi, shiitake, turkey tail, lion's mane, and many others.

Kitchari

Kitchari is part of the traditional Ayurvedic cleanse, Panchakarma. It is high in fiber and protein and full of flavor. This cleanse is great during any season and when liquid cleanses are not suitable. I learned the recipe shared here at an ashram in NYC over twenty years ago. It is traditionally used in Ayurvedic clinics in India. Although curanderismo does not have an equivalent recipe, I know at least three modern curanderas who use this recipe in the same manner as I do. It is a beneficial, nourishing food that helps reset the digestive fire using Ayurvedic elements. Kitchari is a tri-doshic food complementary to the three constitutions defined in Ayurveda as doshas: vata, kapha, and pitta. It is also considered a sattvic food—pure, balanced, and harmonious. Ayurveda considers garlic and onions to be too heating for the digestive system, so these should be avoided not only in kitchari but also in all cooking meant to support wellness. I mention this because, unlike caldo de gallina, where flavor is based on garlic, onions, carrots, and celery, kitchari's flavor derives from the spices used. Spices in the Ayurvedic tradition are the key components to wellness; the powdered spices are equivalent in some cases to the dried herbs we use in Latine herbalism.

For those new to kitchari, the final product should be soft and creamy, with the veggies tender but not mushy, and the spices dancing on the tongue. In Ayurveda, the spices consist of ground herbs, and kitchari presents a means of ingesting these hierbas through food. I find kitchari helpful as a digestive aid when sick and also as a preventative food. Along with my mother, I do a kitchari cleanse twice a year during seasonal shifts to reset digestion from summer to fall and from spring to summer. Changes in weather at these junctures often lead to shifts in the way we eat (as the animals and foods we harvest shift), and this cleanse can prepare our digestive system for these seasonal shifts.

Kitchari Recipe

YIELD: approximately 7 cups fully cooked

1 cup mung lentils (traditional) or split red lentils

¾ cup white basmati rice (traditional) or white jasmine rice

6 cups distilled water

1 cup carrots, sweet potatoes, pumpkin, or other hard vegetables

2 tablespoons ghee

1 teaspoon turmeric powder

1 teaspoon cumin seeds, or ½ teaspoon powdered cumin

1 teaspoon mustard seeds, or ½ teaspoon mustard powder

1 teaspoon fenugreek powder

½ teaspoon asafetida powder

1 teaspoon salt or more to taste

1 cup chopped leafy greens (spinach, kale, mustard greens, etc.), peas, broccoli, or other soft vegetables

¼ cup chopped cilantro

Prepare the lentils by rinsing them three times and soaking them overnight. Rinse the rice until the water runs clear. In a large pot, add the water, rice, and lentils. Bring to a boil, and remove the white foam that arises after 5–10 minutes. When the foam no longer resurfaces, lower the heat to medium and add the harder vegetables, stirring occasionally and checking the tenderness of the lentils and rice. Cook approximately 30 minutes until the mixture reaches a cooked tenderness. Lower to a simmer. There should be about ¼ inch water above the kitchari at this point; if not, add a layer of hot water.

In a separate pan, prepare the spices. Warm the ghee over medium heat and add all the spices except the cilantro, stirring for a few minutes as they become fragrant, but do not overcook. Slowly pour the mixture into the cooked kitchari—it will sizzle, so be careful! Mix and add the softer vegetables. Simmer 5–10 minutes or until the water level is at the top of the mixture. Add the chopped cilantro, remove from heat, and cover for 5 minutes. Using a wire whisk at this stage can help release the lentils' starch and further bind it to the rice, making it easier to digest and assimilate.

Suggested Serving:

- *As a cleanse:* Eat 8- to 10-ounce servings three or four times a day for three days during seasonal changes. If you make a kitchari daily, the choice of vegetables can change each day.
- *For nourishment:* Eat a 10- to 12-ounce portion once a day at lunchtime as well as your regular diet and meals.
- *For use as a preventative:* Choose a three-day time frame each month for a regular cleanse. While fasting works for some, a mono diet of kitchari during these three days can be a welcome relief for your digestion.

FERMENTS

All traditional cuisines have a way of preserving food, not only for a longer shelf life but also for the preventative care of the digestive system. This method of preservation relies on yeast and bacteria to convert sugars and carbohydrates into more beneficial microorganisms, called probiotics, that the body can use. Bacteria and flora in the stomach and intestines react positively with these microorganisms. Examples of fermented foods and drinks include cheeses, pickled vegetables, and effervescent liquids such as mead and kombucha. In Latin America, these bubbly drinks are often made with heirloom corn, cacao, or fruit. Today, probiotics have become a must-have for a healthy gut. Glancing through the probiotic section of any health market, you will find it filled with liquid probiotic drinks and specialized yogurts—and they are some of the most expensive supplements in the store! I am very proud of the many ancestral recipes that serve as alternatives you can make for yourself. Here are two easy-to-make recipes.

Ancestral Kombucha ✿ *Tepache*

"Tepache" is difficult to translate, but some call it Mexican kombucha. I had this refreshing drink for the first time in my twenties—it was both tart and sweet and smelled a little like cheese. I wasn't impressed. But in my thirties, I had the privilege of visiting a *pueblo mágico* (magic town), Tepoztlán, home to a *tepachería* (tepache brewery) that makes over twenty flavors of tepache. Each was distinct in its flavor, although they all share the same base recipe. Here I share the base recipe made with pineapple rinds. It is important to use organic pineapples, as we will be using the pineapple rind, and organic farming practices preclude the use of harsh chemicals.

Pineapple Tepache Recipe

YIELD: approximately 1½ gallons

2 organic pineapples

¼ cup baking soda

water to wash the pineapples

1 gallon distilled water

8 ounces *piloncillo* or *panela* (unrefined cane sugar)

1 cinnamon stick

2 cloves

EQUIPMENT

scrub brush

1 (6-quart) glass jar

wooden spoon

sharp knife

cotton cheesecloth

rubber band or cotton string

cotton sieve

jug or mason jars, for storing

For any ferment, it is important to use the appropriate equipment, as they can be sensitive to yeast, bacteria, and metal. Sanitize any glass or wood equipment by placing it in water at 170°F for at least 30 seconds.

Choose pineapples that are ripe and ready to eat. First, remove the leaf crown by laying the pineapple on its side and holding the body with your nondominant hand. With your other hand, grab the leaf crown at its base and twist away from you. If the pineapple is ripe, it will come right off.

Wash the pineapples with distilled water and a scrub brush; repeat with water and baking soda, rinsing again with distilled water. This will remove any dirt or residue. Peel the pineapples by cutting away the thick outer layer. Store the pineapple fruit in the refrigerator for later consumption. Add the rinds and the distilled water to a glass jar, covering it with the cheesecloth and securing it around the rim of the jug with the rubber band or string.

Leave it in a dark, cool space overnight. On day 2, add the piloncillo (found at any store with Latine products)—it will be solid, but do not grate or chop it; adding it as is helps the yeast and bacteria grow at a slow pace. Replace the fabric cover and store for two more days. On day 3, bubbles should appear. Mix lightly with the wooden spoon. On day 4, mix again; the effervescence and tartness should

piloncillo (top) and panela

be apparent. For more fermentation, leave it for up to two more days. Once the desired tartness is achieved, mix it again, remove the large pieces, and strain the remainder through the cotton sieve into a glass jug or mason jars. Store it in the refrigerator. Left at room temperature, tepache will continue to ferment. You can experiment with it, but always test tepache before consuming it, ensuring that it does not taste bitter. If you see white mold covering the top of the liquid, it's time to discard it.

Suggested Serving: Tepache tastes best cold; serve over ice. If it seems too concentrated, dilute it with water, starting with a ratio of 1 part water to 3 parts tepache. For a delicious probiotic drink, dilute the tepache with tea instead of water or with the agua de jamaica.

Milk Kefir Grains ✿ *Búlgaros*

Sometimes called milk kefir grains, this mixture of beneficial bacteria is used to ferment milk into kefir and is known in Mexico as *búlgaros*—the literal translation of "Bulgarians," after the probiotic strain *Lactobacillus bulgaricus* discovered by the Bulgarian physician and microbiologist, Stamen Gigov Grigorov.

Búlgaros are sold in Mexico as a grain and as *yogur de búlgaros* (Bulgarian yogurt). My mother recalls consuming both during her youth at a famous restaurant/café in Mexico City called Súper Leche (Super Milk), which offered several flavors on the menu to eat on the premises or for takeout.

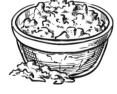

Búlgaros (milk kefir)

In 2023, I finally got to try búlgaros for myself. In Coyoacán (the neighborhood in Mexico City where Frida Kahlo's Casa Azul and museum are located), I spotted an outdoor vendor with a red cooler that bore a sign reading "búlgaros." I jumped for joy to try them, and they did not disappoint. The texture resembled loose cottage cheese, and the flavor was nutty, on the sweet side, and somewhat cheesy. The yogurt was slightly tart, with a medium consistency, and it smelled a bit like umami. This was the first time I tasted búlgaros in my native Mexico, but I have since introduced them to my home in Miami. This is the recipe I share here.

Búlgaros Milk Kefir Recipe

YIELD: 1¼ cups

1 (1.4 grams) dried starter pack or 1 live tablespoon milk kefir grains	1 cup whole milk, room temperature
	fresh fruit (optional)

EQUIPMENT
mason jars
wooden spoon
cotton cheesecloth

rubber band or cotton string
cotton sieve

Búlgaros are not made; they must be cultivated from other grains, just as a vinegar scoby is cultivated from a mother scoby. For this recipe, you will need to purchase the búlgaros—alive or dormant; dormant grains will need extra time to activate (Etsy is a good source)—and follow the seller's instructions for awakening them; usually a one- or two-day process.

Next, to cultivate the grains, place 1–2 tablespoons of búlgaros in the mason jar and add 1 cup of the milk. Cover it with the cheesecloth and secure it around the rim with the rubber band. Store in a warm, dark place for two to four days, checking the ferment every day. You can sample the kefir using the wooden spoon and check for your desired ferment grade. As with tepache, ferments should be tart and cheesy smelling but not stinky or moldy. After some trial and error, you will find the right taste for you. Once you have achieved this, strain the resultant yogurt through the cotton sieve into a bowl for later consumption, making sure not to overly squeeze or shift the búlgaros. The yogurt will be runny and easily digestible, unlike the gooey version sold in the stores.

Transfer the búlgaros to a sterilized mason jar to begin again. They will remain active as long as this cultivating process continues and will reproduce in quantity; at some point, you might want to eat them or gift them. I have found that covering the búlgaros with just enough milk keeps them alive but slows down the reproduction process. Also, the warmer the temperature they are stored in, the faster they reproduce. If you need to pause the cultivation process, store the búlgaros in the refrigerator. When you are ready to awaken them, return them to room temperature, drain, and begin the cultivation process from the start.

Suggested Serving: Drink kefir as is, blend with fruit for a probiotic smoothie, or add to regular smoothies. Búlgaros and kefir are preventative remedios. It is best to drink them weekly for gut health and a smoothly functioning digestive system. It is also a helpful remedio for boosting microorganisms in the aftermath of loose stools, food poisoning, and indigestion.

For a dairy-free alternative: Replace the búlgaros, or milk kefir grains, with water kefir grains, and replace the milk with coconut water.

RITUALS—*RITUALES*

Regarding rituales for the digestive system in curanderismo, we use the word *empacho* (indigestion)—but beyond indigestion, it refers to lack of appetite, a sickly disposition, and someone who is a picky eater. Empacho also infers indigestion that seems to stem from vibrational (mental or emotional) issues such as susto, *berrinche* (tantrum), and mal de ojo. Children are especially susceptible to empacho. Here, I share three very simple rituals that can be used for both adults and children. These rituals represent a modern version of the traditional practice.

Basin Herb Bath ✿ *Baño de hierbas*

Herb baths, often called basin baths or *baño de palangana,* are a common "prescription" by curanderas/os. The use of water and plants dates back to Mesoamerican times. We have only to look at the use of plant baths as rituals by Amazonian tribes of South America to know there is an ancestral link. Herb baths are used to cleanse the vibrational body and, in turn, relieve empacho. I use the ingredients and process I was taught by my father, customizing the hierbas as needed. Prepare by taking a shower, then proceed to the ritual—usually in the bathroom unless you have an outdoor shower, which can be a wonderful experience. The herbs and flowers chosen for this empacho ritual are specific to promoting digestive movement in the physical body and to clear stagnant energy from the vibrational body.

large basin or 3-gallon bucket

2 handfuls fresh *hierba buena* (mint leaves)

¼ cup sea salt

hot water to fill ¼ of the basin

warm water to fill the remaining ¾ of the basin

¼ cup *agua de azahar* (orange blossom water found in the baking isle in Latine groceries)

towel

First, prepare the bath. Add the hierba buena, salt, and hot water to the basin or bucket. Let it steep for 15–30 minutes. Add the remainder of the water and the agua de azahar. Next, standing or sitting on the towel, pick some herbs from the water and rub them on your body, starting at your feet and moving up toward your heart. Once there is only water left in the basin, splash it over your body and pour the last bit over your head. You can sing or play devotional music during the ritual, although prayers are traditional. Air-drying is recommended, or pat dry with a towel, keeping as much of the baño on the skin as possible. After this refreshing ritual, rest is recommended.

Dew Water ❀ *Agua de sereno*

This simple ritual comes from a family friend from the Cuban lineage of curanderismo. The Cuban curandersimo is heavily influenced by Spaniard customs, I have found there are still curanderas/os in the South of Spain that work with *sereno* (dew), collected in the morning from flowers. This is an interesting detail as the famed Bach Flower Remedies created by Doctor Edward Bach were originally made by this very method. Sereno is considered cool and damp; it makes sense from the qualities used in Latine herbalism that this ritual would alleviate the heat of indigestion and empacho.

  pinch of baking soda
  1 glass of water, spring or purified preferred
  3 small white flowers, any flower type

Add the baking soda to the glass of water, mixing well. Add the flowers and place the glass outside at sunset. Leave it uncovered overnight, ensuring that the glass receives morning dew and the first rays of sunrise. Immediately upon awakening, remove the flowers and drink the water on an empty stomach. This ritual is performed for three consecutive days. The result should be a lightness and coolness in the belly.

Lemon Sweep ✿ *Barrida de limón*

The fresh and stimulating aroma of lemons is the key to this ritual. Barridas form the core of curanderismo limpias. They are performed for all ailments, whether physical or energetic. Limpias can be done with hierbas or *flores* (flowers), or a mixture of both. There is no rule as to which herbs and flowers to use, as each curandera/o intuitively finds what works best for each ailment. Also, the available hierbas and flores will vary by region. In general, a barrida is done by forming a bouquet of hierbas and flores and sweeping it over the entire body. In the traditional version, the curandera/o prays over the person while performing the barrida. For those of us who do not follow a religion, mantras, positive affirmations, or devotional music are excellent substitutes. The intention of the barrida is to clear away stagnant energy, allowing for a deeper connection between the physical and vibrational body. The following barrida functions as a natural aromatherapy remedio.

2 whole lemons

¼ cup alcohol

red ribbon or soft belt

Rub each lemon between your hands a few times, gently squeezing. Then roll them across your thigh until they become fragrant. Dip the lemons in the alcohol and rub them all over your body. Continue to roll, dip, and rub until you feel the lifting of stagnant energy. If you are doing this for yourself, ask a friend or family member to rub the back of your body as well. If two lemons are not sufficient, use more as needed. When you are finished, tie the ribbon or belt around your midsection, covering the belly button. Wash your hands and rest. Although simple, this ritual can be a bit heavy as the scent of lemon and use of alcohol raises both body temperature and blood pressure a bit. Make sure to rest and integrate—you will feel refreshed and focused afterward.

————————

A note on all rituals: The herbs and plant materials used in the rituals are meant to be composted after use. You can also bury them in a planter or discard them.

CHAPTER 6

ENERGÍA DE LA LUNA—MOON ENERGY

In the past eight years of working one-on-one with clients, I have observed the benefits of a calm and quiet mind. It allows for a positive outlook, a clear mental process, and better decision-making. Mindfulness practices, meditation techniques, and some forms of yoga have long reflected the maxim that "quiet time equals a quiet mind." In the wellness industry today, we have moved into a space recognizing the importance, beyond a quiet mind, of a regulated nervous system. A quick survey of social media with the hashtag #regulatednervoussystem yields over five thousand posts, attesting to the topic's popularity. Many of my peers in the healing arts rely on valued plants as remedios to calm the nervous system. In curanderismo, we use the term *nervina/o* (nervine; to calm the nerves) for the category of plants that connect to and support the nervous system, specifically to reduce nervous energy.

But what exactly is a calm nervous system? I find that the way our ancestors engaged with *la luna* (the moon) mirrors a regulated nervous system. When the sun sets and the moon rises, the energy is soft, cool, and quiet—unlike when the sun rises, and the energy is dynamic and expansive. In my experience, the energy that results from bathing under the moonlight fosters contemplation, patience, and a dreamy state of mind. A regulated nervous system is one that integrates and reflects these qualities.

One way I promote this metaphoric lunar energy with my clients is through the following meditation:

Find a comfortable spot and sit, placing your hands on your lap.

Breathe in the cool air, visualizing this air moving into your spine.

Breathe out, visualizing this cool air expanding in your spine.

After a few breaths, focus on just the air at the spine, slowly converting it to an iridescent pearl-white color.

Continue to breathe and concentrate on this visual for 10–20 breaths.

Rub your hands softly and place them over your eyes for 4 breaths.

Lower your hands and open your eyes slowly.

The feedback I receive speaks to how this meditation changes people's body temperature. It quiets their thoughts and completely relaxes their bodies. These are some of the benefits of encouraging moon energy in the body.

La luna, according to many traditional spiritual philosophies, is linked to the dream state. For most of us, a normal rhythm is to be awake during the daytime and asleep at night. The dream state, which reveals itself only during sleep, is thus evoked in the nocturnal phase. Our notions about the moon and nocturnal sleep as a time when magic and the creative imagery of dreams can be called upon have inspired moonlit rites and rituals over the centuries, linking dreams and magic with la luna.

Curanderismo and the moon are old friends. Rituals with Mesoamerican roots include moon dances, crystal gazing, and moonlight plant baths. The teachings from my family lineage in curanderismo represent a blend of Western beliefs adopted during colonization. For example, the belief that la luna can induce temporary madness is reflected in the term *lunática/o* (lunatic), derived from the Latin word for "moonstruck." This belief was brought by colonization and is not native to the Mesoamerican Indigenous, who viewed *el sol* (sun) as a father to Mother Earth and la luna as a grandmother. La luna was gentle; her moonbeams were subtle yet strong enough to light the darkness. She was a protector who kept our ancestors, the stars, under her watchful eye.

It is said in my home that emotions intensify during a *luna llena* (full moon), making it important to treat others kindly. It is also a time to harness lunar energy and accomplish important tasks. I believe that lunar energy creates a low-grade electromagnetic field that heightens our own personal human magnetic field, and that any significant tasks, remedios, and rituales performed during this time become infused with amplified energy. Be aware that all energies are heightened, including the negative ones. If you choose to work with a luna llena, be aware of this and approach your remedios y rituales with positive intentions. Limpias under the full moon are especially powerful. The amplification of energy results in potent release of stagnant and unwanted vibrations.

REMEDIES—*REMEDIOS*

The remedios in this chapter will address regulating the nervous system, connecting to the dream state, and influencing mental states. Plant allies in these categories are pungent in their aroma and are used both orally and topically. I have discovered that once you connect to a particular hierba, it becomes a much-loved and utilized plant in your herbolaria and a favorite remedio on your wellness journey.

Chamomile Tea ❧ *Té de manzanilla*

Chamomile (*L. Chamomilla recutita*)—*Manzanilla*
ENERGY: Cold/dry | TASTE: Bitter | PLANT PART USED: Flower, stem, leaf

This tea is one that all *abuelitas* (grandmas) make when children can't sleep. It is also one of the first teas given to children when they begin to drink water-based liquids. For Latine adults, chamomile tea can be very comforting, awakening memories of childhood. A strong tea is made using the stems, leaves, and flowers of the hierba. In Latine markets, you will find the plant material uncut, dried, and folded into cellophane bags for sale. In herbal dispensaries, you might find merely flowers and stems; either are good choices as tea substances.

Chamomile Tea Recipe

YIELD: approximately 2 cups

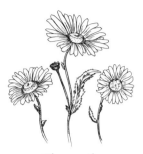

Chamomile

> 2 tablespoons chamomile hierba
> 2 cups water
> preferred sweetener

In a French press, add hot water (just boiled) to the hierbas, cover, and steep for 4 hours. Strain and serve.

Suggested Use: Drink 1 cup 30 minutes before bedtime or to induce sleep at any time.

- *Adults:* Use 1 part tea concentrate to 1 part hot water.
- *Children over 7:* Use 1 part tea concentrate to 3 parts warm water.
- *Children under 7 and infants:* Use 1 part tea concentrate to 9 parts warm water for sleep and colic.
- *Optional:* Use as a digestive aid for stomach pain, loose bowels, and flatulence. Serve as a substitute for té de menta (page 99).

Cannabis or CBD Alcohol Rub ❀
Alcohol de canabis o CBD

Cannabis (*L. Cannabis sativa*)—*Canabis*

ENERGY: Cold/damp | PLANT PART USED: Bud

Cannabis is used in Mexico recreationally, as in many other countries. While it is not a native plant, I have had discussions with healers in Oaxaca who use marijuana in place of a difficult-to-find plant called *pipiltzintzintli (L. Salvia divinorum)*, which is used for ancestral dreaming and as a hallucinogen in healing rituals. Cannabis sativa seems to hold that energy for them. For our use, the CBD bud adequately induces la luna energy of relaxation.

A short walk from Mexico City's Metropolitan Cathedral in *El Zócalo* (La Plaza de la Constitución) gives way to a street where you can buy all kinds of remedios herbarios. Vendors line up on the street with their artisanal preparaciónes, largely made with herbs they grow themselves. Among the many remedios and hierbas to browse through, one amazing preparación herbaria is an infused alcohol made with cannabis. Alcohol rubs in Mexico are popular with the Indigenous and are made with aguardiente (sugarcane alcohol). They are similar to tinctures but are not meant to be ingested. I remember my grandfather rubbing his body with alcohol before bed, but I wasn't sufficiently curious to ask why until my aunt began rubbing my grandmother with alcohol in her geriatric life stage. This is called a *friega de alcohol* (alcohol massage). The alcohol was infused, just like a tincture, with an herb called *axihuitl* (*L. Ageratina pichinchensis*), which acts as a pain reliever.

I have experienced alcohol rubbings several times, and they are not nearly as comforting as a massage. The first thing we need to understand is that the intent of the friega is to make you sweat. The alcohol is initially cold as it evaporates and then turns the skin hot, opening the pores. This cold and hot friction is meant to jumpstart a temperature switch that will (1) absorb the herbal properties through the hot phase, and (2) heat the body to the point of sweating and/or relieving pain. Either way, the friega with infused alcohol is a deeply relaxing and pain-relieving rub.

Cannabis or CBD Alcohol Rub Recipe

YIELD: approximately 2 cups

1 cup CBD herbs or medicinal cannabis herbs	mason jar
	cotton sieve
2 cups aguardiente, vodka, or isopropyl alcohol	1 (4-ounce) amber mist jar

Add the hierba and the alcohol to the mason jar, mixing well. Leave it in a cool, dark place for a full lunar cycle, starting and ending at the full moon. Decant and strain through the cotton sieve into a clean jar for storing, squeezing the hierba to release all of its properties. Dispense into the mist bottle for topical use.

Suggested Use: For adults only. Spray and rub infused alcohol into the chest before bedtime. Cover the chest with a loose, cotton shirt to contain the heat and warm the body.

Valerian Tincture ❃ *Tintura de valeriana*

Valerian (*L. Valeriana officinalis*)—*Valeriana*

ENERGY: Hot/dry | TASTE: Pungent | PLANT PART USED: Root

Valerian root is another hierba introduced by the Spaniards. This aromatic plant can induce relaxation in smaller quantities and deep sleep in larger quantities. Because the taste is so pungent, it is best taken as a tincture in water or another liquid. The root can be purchased at herb dispensaries and is usually cut and sifted, ready for use. It can be blended with chamomile or lavender for a more effective formula and palatable flavor.

Valerian Tincture Recipe

YIELD: approximately 1 cup

½ cup valerian root

1 cup vodka or agua ardiente

small (1-pint) mason jars

cotton sieve

1 (2-ounce) amber dropper bottle

Place the valerian root and vodka in a mason jar, mixing well. Seal it tightly and place it in a cool, dark spot for a full lunar cycle. Strain it through the cotton sieve, squeezing the hierba as you strain. Store the tincture in a clean mason jar and dispense it into the dropper bottle for use.

Suggested Use: This tincture can be fast-acting due to the body's rapid absorption of alcohol.

- *For relaxation:* Take half a dropper with liquid. Wait 4 hours between dosages.
- *For sleeping:* Take 1 full dropper 30 minutes before bedtime. If this is insufficient, take 2 droppers the following evening, but avoid taking more than one dose in a single evening. Be sure to schedule 6–8 hours of sleep and be ready to rest when taking.

Lavender Salve ❀ *Pomada de lavanda*

Lavender (*L. Lavandula angustifolia*)—*Lavanda*

ENERGY: Cold/dry | PLANT PART USED: Buds

Lavender salve is a preparación herbaria that should be in everyone's herbolaria. It not only supports relaxation but can also be used for its antibacterial properties on cuts, blisters, or other skin eruptions. Lavender salve is gentle enough for children and infants in small quantities and can also be used for diaper rash. I often carry a lavender-chamomile-peppermint balm in my purse to counter low-grade anxiety and a nervous stomach. Plus, I find the aroma quite comforting.

Lavender Salve Recipe

YIELD: approximately 9 ounces

1 cup coconut oil

½ cup dried lavender buds

mason jar

1 ounce candelilla wax

12 drops lavender essential oil

1 (2-ounce) metal tin

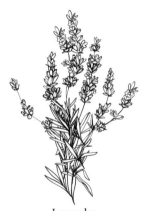

Lavender

Infuse the coconut oil with the lavender buds in the mason jar, following the instructions for Oil Infusion (page 35). Next, melt the wax in a double boiler and slowly add the infused oil. The wax will harden slightly; warm the mixture until the wax melts again and let it combine for 15 minutes. Turn off the heat and wait 2–5 minutes for the peak heat to reduce. Transfer the mixture back to the mason jar, add the essential oil, and stir well. Dispense the salve into the metal tin for storage and use. For a softer texture, follow the instructions for Basic Preparation for Balms, Salves, and Ointments (page 43).

Suggested Use: Apply to the chest and the soles of the feet. Use liberally and gently massage it in for complete absorption. For a relaxing experience, draw a warm footbath, adding lavender and chamomile hierbas. Soak your feet for 15–20 minutes, dry them, and apply the lavender salve. Wear socks to aid absorption and help warm the body.

Linden Syrup ❀ *Jarabe de tilo*

Linden (*L. Tilia cordata* or *Tilia platyphyllos*)—*Tilo*

ENERGY: Cold/damp | **PLANT PART USED:** Flower, leaf

Regarding *hierbas calmantes* (calming herbs), there is either team chamomile or team linden. It is said in Mexico that the working class uses *manzanilla* (chamomile) and the upper class uses *tilo* (linden). Chamomile continues to be farmed in the

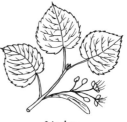

Linden

pueblos and harvested when it flowers, while linden is harvested in the tree stage and sourced from herb dispensaries. For relaxation, I prefer chamomile, reserving linden for dreamwork. Many clients have reported vivid dreams after taking linden at bedtime; some have reported sleepwalking. Linden contains a natural form of a benzodiazepine-like compound that can induce a more hypnotic than relaxed state in some people. Linden syrup is meant for deep sleep—when you want to remember your dreams and let the subconscious work itself out in the dream state.

Linden Syrup Recipe

YIELD: approximately 1 cup

½ cup linden hierba, cut and sifted

1 cup water

¼ cup sweetener of choice

¼ cup brandy

small (1-pint) mason jar

1 (4-ounce) pour bottle

Prepare the tea according to the recipe for Water Infusion (page 34), with a 6-hour steep time. Add the sweetener to the warm tea, letting it dissolve completely. When it reaches room temperature, add the brandy and stir well. Pour it into the mason jar and store it in the refrigerator. Dispense into the pour bottle for use. The brandy and sweetener can be substituted with sweet white wine.

Suggested Use: Begin with 1 tablespoon before bedtime, or 2 tablespoons if sleep eludes you. Find the right dose for entering a dream state. Keep a journal by your bedside for morning notes when you awaken. Jarabe de tilo can be used in conjunction with the obsidian-gazing ritual in the next section.

RITUALS—*RITUALES*

The rituals in this section are largely for dreamwork. La luna energy enhances the connection to the dream state. Try these rituals during a full moon and keep track of the imagery. A good symbolism or totem book will help you find meaning in your subconscious dreams.

Obsidian Mirror ❋ *Espejo de obsidiana*

I bought my first *tezcatl* (obsidian mirror) in Teotihuacán, a prehistoric Mesoamerican city considered to be one of the largest cities of the ancient Americas. Today, it is a historic site where visitors can tour the vast, expansive ruins. As is common at tourist spots, many vendors sell their artisanal goods and tell the stories behind them. The vendor I bought my obsidian mirror from shared the following with me:

> The name "tezcatl" was derived from the Aztec deity Tezcatlipoca. He was the deity ruling over the nocturnal sky. His name meant "smoking mirror," as he is often depicted with an obsidian mirror on his body, and it is said he used the smoke of hallucinogenic hierbas to bring himself into a trance before looking into the obsidian mirror. Gazing into the mirror can conjure visions of the underworld, access the ancestral realm, and tap into the subconscious.

As I contemplated whether to purchase it, I asked him to show me how to use it. He said it was used only at night, amid the soft reflection of candlelight or *rayos de luna* (moonbeams). I have used this obsidian mirror as a protective amulet many times and twice to view solar eclipses, shielding my eyes, but only a handful of times as a gazing mirror. It is a practice that requires dedication and time, with results that can be quite wondrous when refined. In Europe, the practice of gazing into mirrored surfaces is called "scrying." How interesting it is to see the connection of customs between cultures.

I also share with you the ritual of *sahumar* (smudging). This is another important limpia in curanderismo. Since pre-Columbian times, ceremonial smudging has traditionally been performed with copal, or copalli, a word of Nahuatl origin, meaning "incense." Copal is also a resin from the Burseraceae variety tree (*L. Protium copal*). Today, copal incense is best known for its use during the Día de los Muertos (Day of the Dead) festivities. The folklore around copal mentions its use as an offering in which the smoke carries our gratitude, petitions, and prayers to the ancestral realms. The traditional method for this ritual incorporates a special smudging vessel called a *copalera* (incense vessel), charcoal bricks, and copal resin in its natural form. In Mexico, these items can be found at specialty markets year-round; in the USA, they can be located at Latine shops during the Day of the Dead season. Incorporating copal resin with obsidian mirror-gazing supports relaxation and the opening of the subconscious.

Obsidian Mirror Ritual

copalera

incense charcoal and lighter

copal resin incense

large 5- to 8-inch obsidian mirror

journal and pencil

Choose a night with a luna llena and find comfortable seating outdoors. Light the charcoal in the copalera and begin burning the copal incense, letting the smoke flow with the wind. Place the obsidian mirror at an angle on a surface in front of you, finding the reflection of the moon. Sit with your feet flat on the floor, barefoot if possible, with a straight spine. Close your eyes and take 10 long, slow breaths, focusing on quieting the mind. Slowly open your eyes, keeping your gaze downward on the obsidian mirror. Allow your eyes to focus in and out while breathing slowly; let your mind wander. The results of the ritual will vary, depending on what your inquiry might be. In general, if you partake in this ritual with a positive state of mind and an open heart, the subconscious mind will reveal areas in your life that can be nurtured with love, compassion, and joy. To complete the ritual, close your eyes again and take several deep breaths, contemplating any information that was revealed. Open your eyes; journal about your thoughts and conclusions. Take a cool shower to restore your vibrational body to normal before going to sleep.

Dreamtime Ritual ✿ *Ritual del sueño*

I learned about *artemisa* (mugwort) from one of my folk herbalism teachers in NYC, who spoke of its sedative qualities. Mugwort has the reputation, in both curanderismo and Traditional Western Herbalism, of inducing lucid dreams and bringing on a hypnotic state, similar to linden. It can be used as a tea, an incense, and an herbal smoke inhalant.

Dreamtime Ritual Method

small cotton muslin bag
¼ cup organic mugwort
journal and pencil

For this ritual, choose any point in the lunar phase, but be sure to schedule sufficient hours of sleep afterward. This usage of mugwort will induce more sleep than you might be used to. Mugwort is pungent; even in a cotton bag, it will leave its scent behind. Keep this dreamtime amulet away from all pets and children.

Add the mugwort to the bag and close it tightly. At bedtime, rub the bag between your hands, warming it as you do so. Set the intention to remember your dreams, and place the bag on the pillow, next to your head. Focus on the aroma and take deep breaths. You will be asleep before you know it. When you awaken, before beginning your day, take some time to journal about any observations and dreams you recall.

Optional: Make a dreamtime balm following the Lavender Salve Recipe on page 81, replacing the lavender with mugwort. Apply it to your temples before sleeping.

CHAPTER 7

VIBRACIÓN DEL ALIENTO—ESSENCE OF THE BREATH

Breath is the one physical process of the body we cannot live without. If we stop breathing, we stop living. It is imperative that the breath flow in its natural state for as long as possible. While breathing can be manipulated, as in deep, conscious breaths, it can also occur automatically, as it does during sleep. It can be easy to forget the importance of breath until we lack its effortless flow. I have personally struggled with breathing since childhood; many times, I was put on oxygen tanks and nebulizers to open my lungs. It was not until I moved to Miami at the age of nine and had a tonsillectomy that my breathing became normal.

In curanderismo, the lungs are kept healthy by administering stimulating hierba remedies that promote the opening of the breath. The chosen remedy depends on the specific area of stagnation: when the breath is stagnant in the nasal passages, we apply the remedio via the nose using a liquid wash or inhalants; if the breath is stagnant in the throat, as with coughing, the remedio can range from inhalants to teas to topical rubs. Stagnation in the lungs can improve with topical rubs.

From a vibrational standpoint, similar to the beliefs held by other schools of traditional herbal folk wellness, the lungs are said to hold disappointment, sadness, and grief. In addition to the death toll of the COVID pandemic, 2020 marked many endings on a global scale. My response was to offer rituales that support the release of our emotions. While endings can also be beginnings, my experience is that *all* endings with transformative results need to be grieved—whether it is a lost job, a divorce, or a move to another state. The rituals in this chapter are condensed versions of larger ones. I hope they will soothe your heart in times of grief and support your life experience for easy and flowing breath.

REMEDIES—*REMEDIOS*

Cinnamon Tea ✿ *Té de canela*

Cinnamon (*L. Cinnamomum cassia*)—*Canela*

ENERGY: Hot/dry | **TASTE:** Sweet | **PLANT PART USED:** Bark

Cinnamon in Mexico is a different variety than the type sold in the USA. If you purchase the stick version in Mexico, you might notice it has multiple layers and a flaky exterior. This is typically Ceylon cinnamon—grown, sold, and also used in India, Bali, and other parts of Southeast Asia—native to Sri Lanka. The variety commonly found in the USA is Cassia cinnamon, native to China and other parts of East Asia; it has a thicker, harder stick with no layers. For our purposes, either of these varieties is fine; their therapeutic properties are similar.

Cinnamon is considered hot in its herbal energetics. It should be used with caution because too much heat in the body can lead to temporarily elevated blood pressure, headaches, and internal dryness. Because of this, I also offer an atole version of this tea so it can benefit both a dry and a wet stagnation of the breath.

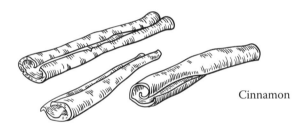

Cinnamon

Cinnamon Tea Recipe

1 (2-inch) cinnamon stick

2 cups water

preferred sweetener

Place the cinnamon and the water in a pot. Bring to a boil and simmer, covered, for 10 minutes. Strain and serve. Add sweetener if desired.

Suggested Use: For a wet cough that manifests as phlegm and mucus in the nose, throat, and lungs. Drink 1 cup every 4–6 hours.

Cinnamon Atole ❀ *Atole de canela*

ENERGY: Hot/dry | **TASTE:** Sweet

Atol, Atole, *Atolli,* or *Atol de Elote* is a traditional drink of many Latin American Indigenous cultures. Stemming from the Nahuatl word for "watery," this corn-based drink with pre-Hispanic roots is used in both celebration and gratitude. Modern additives such as cacao, herbs, and fruit enhance the original concoction of dry, ground maíz and water. This drink contains carbohydrates, fat, and protein. Maíz is an easily digestible starch that acts as both a pre- and probiotic, helping to absorb food nutrients more efficiently; fruit and cacao increase absorption even further while leaving us feeling more satisfied for longer.

While cinnamon is hot and dry, the maíz in the atole works to moisten. Because of this, cinnamon atole is good for dry ailments of the respiratory system—including dry sinuses, cough, tight chest, itchy throat, and pneumonia or bronchitis with a dry cough. This drink is warming, nourishing, and decadent. It can be prepared with vanilla extract for added flavor. This recipe blends my mother's version using *masa harina* (corn flour used for making tortillas) with slippery elm powder for gut health and extra moistening of the digestive tract.

Cinnamon Atole Recipe

1 cup Cinnamon Tea (page 91)

1 tablespoon slippery elm powder (*L. Ulmus rubra*)

2 tablespoons masa harina

½ teaspoon cinnamon powder

1 teaspoon vanilla extract (optional)

sweetener to taste

In a small bowl, mix 1 or 2 tablespoons of the tea with the slippery elm powder until a paste is formed. Add the cinnamon and masa harina to a pot and "flash roast" it on low heat until it becomes more yellow-hued and less cream-colored. Slowly add the remaining cinnamon tea, stirring briskly until the flour is fully incorporated and all lumps are dissolved. Continue stirring until you see a few bubbles. Remove it from the heat and add the vanilla extract (optional) and the slippery elm paste. Blend well and add sweetener to taste.

Suggested Use: Drink 1 cup every 3–4 hours. When actively sick, drink this before each meal to support the digestion of food while warming the body and calming the cough. It can also be used as a preventative at the first sign of a cold or flu.

Holy Wood Tea ❧ *Té de palo santo*

Palo santo (*L. Bursera graveolens*)—*Palo santo*

ENERGY: Cooling/dry | **TASTE:** Bitter and astringent | **PLANT PART USED:** Wood and resin

Palo santo (holy wood) is known today for its smudging qualities. As its name implies, it is considered a holy or saintly tree. When a hierba is given the adjective "holy" or "sacred," it is usually because the surrounding folklore points to its repeated success. Palo santo is used as wood, resin, and essential oil. The wood is burned for smudging and steeped as tea. The resin is also used

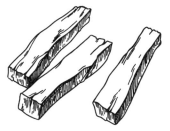
Palo santo

for smudging and for making balms for pain relief. The essential oil is used in various preparaciónes for respiratory ailments, skin eruptions, and insect control.

Palo Santo Tea Recipe

YIELD: approximately 1 cup

2- to 3-inch palo santo wood stick

1 cup water

heatproof cup

preferred sweetener

Bring the water to a boil, then add it to a cup along with the palo santo. Steep for 15–20 minutes. Remove palo santo and serve. Add sweetener if desired.

Suggested Use: For a wet cough with fever. Drink 1 cup every 2–4 hours. Note the best palo santo for this is the wood with dark color parts, this is the resin in the wood that is both aromatic and therapeutic.

Holy Herb Syrup ✿ *Jarabe de yerba santa*

Holy herb (*L. Eriodictyon californicum*)—*Yerba santa*

ENERGY: Hot/dry | TASTE: Sweet and earthy | PLANT PART USED: Leaf and resin

I have witnessed the healing effects of this botanical—another "holy" hierba known for its respiratory support. Yerba santa cuts through mucus and phlegm incredibly well, but, as with cinnamon, it should be used with caution due to its heating qualities. Yerba santa can also be made as a tea, following the instructions for Water Infusion (page 34). The suggested steep time is 1–2 hours; dilute with equal parts tea and water to serve.

Holy Herb Syrup Recipe

½ cup yerba santa hierba, cut

½ cup linden hierba, cut and sifted

2 cloves

2 cups water

1 cup honey or maple syrup

¼ cup brandy or jerez

mason jar

Mix the yerba santa, linden, cloves, and water in a pot; bring it to a boil and steep for 4 hours. Strain well and add the honey or maple syrup, letting it dissolve completely. When the mixture reaches room temperature, add the brandy or jerez and mix well. Store in the mason jar in the refrigerator for up to two weeks.

Suggested Use: Not recommended for children.

- *For adolescents:* 1 tablespoon every 4 hours.
- *For adults:* Begin with 1 tablespoon and increase the dose up to 2 tablespoons, as needed. The linden properties in this syrup will support relaxation and respiratory relief.
- *Optional:* Chamomile or lavender can replace the linden.

Garlic Honey Vinegar ❁
Tónico de vinagre y ajo con miel

Garlic (*L. Allium sativum*)—*Ajo*

ENERGY: Hot/dry | TASTE: Bitter and astringent | PLANT PART USED: Bulb

Honey—*Miel*

ENERGY: Cold/moist | TASTE: Sweet

Vinegar—*Vinagre*

ENERGY: Hot/dry | TASTE: Acidic and astringent

Infused vinegars have surged in popularity in recent years. Wellness advocates pushed for a morning shot of vinegar for preventative purposes. In Mexico, however, vinegars are used sparingly, even for culinary purposes, as they are known to overstimulate the digestive system. I believe their use should be restricted to remedio purposes on an as-needed basis. Vinegar helps open the respiratory passages with its pungent, camphor-like vapors, in addition to its hot and drying properties.

Garlic has been used as a cure-all in Mexico since its introduction in the seventeenth century. Its subtle therapeutic properties make it suitable for both culinary and preventative purposes. I have met many Mexicans who swear that eating one garlic clove a day will keep you free of any flu, cold, or parasitic ailments. Whether true or not, I know firsthand that garlic, as a natural expectorant and antimicrobial hierba, can cut through mucus and phlegm quickly. Interestingly, garlic is also revered for its use in vibrational limpias. These are prepared with aguardiente and applied through *sopladas* (oral water blowing). In Guatemala, this ritual was performed on me by an incredible healer. In this particular limpia, the curandera/o chews the garlic, mixes it with a shot of aguardiente in their mouth, and blows away the stagnant energy from the recipient's body. This ritual left me feeling purified, and all stagnant energy was released.

Honey is used in many cultures for its antimicrobial properties, both on the skin and internally. Because it carries the same density and mineral content as blood, it is used in Ayurveda to increase vitality and prana (life force) in the body. I use it in this recipe for its antimicrobial and sweetening properties.

Garlic Honey Vinegar Recipe

YIELD: approximately 1½ cups

mortar and pestle	1 cup honey
6 peeled garlic cloves	½ cup apple cider vinegar or
mason jar	pineapple vinegar

Crush the garlic cloves in the mortar and pestle until they pop open—no need to crush too hard. Place them in the mason jar with the honey and mix well, making sure to incorporate any garlic juices. Add the vinegar and mix again. The tonic will be runny in consistency. Store it in the refrigerator for up to a week, checking that the mixture does not develop a skin or a smell akin to wet socks. If this happens, compost or discard the mixture; it is a sign of mold. Alternatively, infuse the vinegar with the garlic cloves for one week before mixing in the honey.

Suggested Use: This tónico is especially comforting when there is coughing with phlegm and for sinus infections. When actively sick, take 1 tablespoon every 2 hours. If you are brave, take a shot every 4 hours. Not recommended for children under ten years.

Leo's Remedy ❀ *Remedio de Papi*

Orange (*L. Citrus sinensis*)—*Naranja de china*

ENERGY: Hot/dry | TASTE: Sweet | PART USED: Juice

Ginger (*L. Zingiber officinale*)—*Jengibre*

ENERGY: Hot/dry | TASTE: Spicy and pungent | PART USED: Root

Garlic (*L. Allium sativum*)—Ajo

ENERGY: Hot/dry | **TASTE:** Bitter and astringent | **PLANT PART USED:** Bulb

Honey—*Miel*

ENERGY: Cold/moist | **TASTE:** Sweet

Leo is my father's name, and this is my version of his remedy for opening the throat, lungs, and sinus passages. My father (Papi, to me) was born in the jungles of Cuba. He lived a rustic life and was not vaccinated or introduced to allopathic medicine until he was a teenager. His knowledge of herbs was a natural extension of living in harmony with the land. When I suffered from congestion and breathing ailments, he would administer this elixir—made with 1 cup of fresh ginger boiled in orange juice for 5 minutes—that would bring me to tears. I dreaded this elixir; no amount of honey would stop the burning! Not until my studies of folk herbalism did I understand just how powerful and necessary this remedio was for me. In 2016, he made this elixir for me to

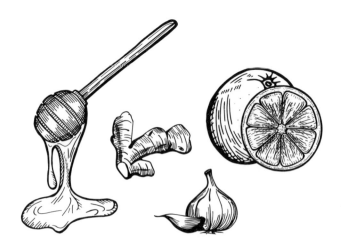

treat chikungunya attacks I was suffering from. This time, I drank it with a smile, and it brought much relief.

Leo's Remedy

YIELD: approximately 1 cup

1 cup orange juice, freshly squeezed

1 tablespoon freshly grated ginger root

2 garlic bulbs, grated

pinch of cinnamon

honey or sweetener to taste

Add the orange juice, ginger, and garlic to a pot and bring it to a boil. Remove it from the heat and let it cool for a few minutes. Strain, add the cinnamon and honey or sweetener, and serve.

Optional: Blend the orange juice, ginger, and garlic together in a blender; transfer it to a pot and heat to a low simmer.

Suggested Use: Drink ¼ cup every 2 hours when you are actively sick. Use as a preventative during cold and flu season.

Peppermint Inhaler ✿ *Inhalador de menta*

Peppermint (*L. Mentha x piperita*)—*Yerba buena*

ENERGY: Cold/dry | TASTE: Bitter | PLANT PART USED: Leaf and stem

Menthol crystal—Cornmint (*L. Mentha arvensis*)—*Crystal de menta*

ENERGY: Cold/dry | PLANT PART USED: Concentrated leaf and stem

In the nineteen years I lived in New York City I spent at least ten winter seasons suffering from debilitating nasal infections.

This inhaler method saved me on many mornings when the stuffiness and pain was at its worst. In the last of those years, I would take the time to steam once every other week as a preventative measure that kept the sinus issues at bay. As plants are powerful any time of the year, I also recommend this recipe during allergy season for those who suffer from stuffy nose and dry cough.

Peppermint Inhaler Recipe

water to fill a basin or large pot ¾ full

medium basin or pot, approximately 10 inches wide

1 small menthol crystal

4 drops peppermint essential oil

2 large towels

In a large pot, bring the water to a boil, let it rest for a minute, and pour it into the basin—or leave it in the pot if a basin is unavailable. Add the menthol crystal and the essential oil drops.

Suggested Use: Use while actively sick. This inhaler can help with allergies, sinus pressure, colds, flu, or any ailment that stagnates the breath in the nasal passages. Place the basin or pot on a flat surface and lean your face over it to breathe in the vapors, covering your head, shoulders, and the basin with the towel, or two, to keep the warmth and steam contained. Keep your eyes closed. If a menthol crystal is inaccessible, it can be omitted.

Vaporu Rub ❀ *Pomada de vaporu*

Peppermint (*L. Mentha x piperita*)—*Yerba buena*

ENERGY: Cold/dry | PLANT PARTS USED: Leaf and stem

Lavender (*L. Lavandula angustifolia*)—*Lavanda*

ENERGY: Cold/dry | PLANT PART USED: Buds

Eucalyptus (*L. Eucalyptus globulus*)—*Eucalipto*

ENERGY: Cool/moist/stimulating | **PLANT PARTS USED:** Leaf

Cedarwood (*L. Juniperus virginiana*)—*Cedro*

ENERGY: Hot/dry/expectorant | **PLANT PARTS USED:** Bark, needles, leaves

Many readers will know exactly what this name refers to, even with the intended typo. For others, it refers to an age-old Vaseline-based commercial balm that our parents and grandparents used to treat coughs, colds, and flu symptoms. I have been making an all-natural alternative for many years. It is the first compound preparación I made in my kitchen, around 2010. Knowing the formula helped, but envisioning a version that was Vaseline (petroleum)-free, I came up with an effective rub that brings both comfort and pain relief. This preparación involves multiple steps; you can make a large batch every season and fine-tune the ingredients once you get the hang of it.

Vaporu Rub Recipe

essential oils blend: 6 drops peppermint, 4 drops lavender, 4 drops eucalyptus, and 2 drops cedarwood

1 gram menthol crystals

2 cups grapeseed oil

½ cup dried lavender buds

2 ounces candelilla or beeswax

1 (16-ounce) amber glass jar for storing 1 (2-ounce) glass jar for dispensing

In a small bowl, dissolve the menthol crystals in the essential oils blend and let it sit uncovered, overnight. In a double boiler, infuse the grapeseed oil with the lavender buds following the instructions for Oil Infusion (page 35). Strain the infused oil and return it to the double boiler; follow the instructions for Basic Preparation for Balms, Salves, and Ointments (page 43) to complete.

Suggested Use: This balm can help relieve symptoms from stagnated energy or respiratory ailments. Rub it on the chest, sides of neck, temples, and forehead. It is customary in curanderismo to also rub the lymphatic meridians: Apply the balm to the inner elbows, armpits, and behind the knees. For extra support, rub it on the soles of the feet and cover with socks.

Optional: Use this balm as a space cleanser. My mother uses a water smudge during times of illness when there is coughing and sneezing. You will need a heat source such as a hot plate, an old small pot, water, and the Vaporu Rub. Place the hot plate in the middle of the room you want to clear. Fill the pot halfway with water and bring it to a boil. Lower it to a simmer and add one tablespoon of the pomada. Let simmer for 10–15 minutes. You can also take the pot to other rooms while the water is hot and steam out any microbes and bacteria.

RITUALS—*RITUALES*

The following rituals are my personal versions of two that are performed at funerals and wakes and for Día de los Muertos (Day of the Dead). They are meant to honor the deceased and expel the energies of grief and sadness. I believe that emotions should be noticed, felt, released, and integrated. The rituals are a process of letting emotions "move out" from a stagnated place or suppression. As a holistic wellness modality, curanderismo holds the belief that mental and emotional states affect overall health.

Emotions that are continually suppressed will eventually make you sick. There is value in "feeling your feelings" to help move the energy of feelings into a space of integration. Grief, in particular, seems to bring up secondary suppressed emotions, making it all the more important to process this emotion to allow for freedom and release.

Devotional Altar ❁ *Ofrenda*

During Día de los Muertos, the word *"ofrenda"* (sacred offering) is used to signify a devotional altar. In the largely Indigenous state of Oaxaca, Mexico, ofrendas range from a small table to entire rooms. Each ofrenda is curated to hold copal, flowers, candles, and images of deceased loved ones—along with their favorite foods, snacks, and *vicios* (vices) while they were alive. I call it a devotional altar because during the three to five days it stays open around this holiday in late October/early November, the family will change out the food, add more flowers, and at times pull up a chair to bring the deceased up to date with family news. The energy of these altars is *alive.* They are interactive altars where the family creates a portal of energy to connect with the deceased.

When I have clients experiencing deep grief, my first question is always, "When was the last time you honored your deceased?" By "honor," I don't mean just thinking about them; thinking about a person who is no longer incarnate without taking any action often leads to a feeling of emptiness and increases the sense of grief. This is the beauty of the ofrenda: it involves an action that allows for a somatic release of the emotion of grief. As the period for ofrendas recurs annually, you know that every year there will be a time for you to sit with your feelings. I find that this type of devotional process acts as a limpia, an emotional cleanse that leaves you lighter and more grounded. There is also a feeling of deep release when you are "allowed" to connect with the ancestors without shame around feelings of grief and sadness.

This ritual is for anyone, at any time of the year, who needs to process grief surrounding a person, a situation, or even a personal objective that has not worked out as expected. It is meant as a personal one-on-one experience and not to be performed for others experiencing grief, although it can be shared with them. As with all altars this ofrenda includes all elemental energies of, Earth, Water, Fire, and Air, along with photographs incorporating images of the deceased, situations, or personal objectives that are mourned.

Devotional Altar Ritual

small table

cloth or shawl

flowers

photographs

copalera

copal resin incense

incense charcoal and lighter

1 small glass of ritual water or holy water (special combination of herbs and flowers in alcohol used for rituals, such as Agua Florida)

1 small bowl of salt

For a person: 1 or more favorite foods of the deceased

For a situation or objective: small objects or other representations that hold meaning for you

journal and pencil

Find a place in your home or garden where you will be able to sit comfortably and set up the ofrenda for seven days without moving it. Drape the table with a beautiful cloth and arrange the flowers, photos, water, salt, and other objects you will be using. Leave space for dishes if you will offer food. Sit at the altar for seven days at the same time every day, ideally, undisturbed by outside demands. Change the water when it evaporates, replace the food items daily, and refresh the flowers as needed.

Begin the ritual by lighting the copalera, letting the smoke purify the space. Place the food on the altar and sit for a few deep breaths. You are invited to talk, cry, sing, or just sit in remembrance. Let the emotions bubble up, let them flow, and know you have set this time to experience your feelings. I find that a good time frame for this ritual is 45 minutes; more, if possible, but it depends entirely on your resilience in moving through the emotions. Once you feel complete with the ritual, journal about your experience to ground the energy before you step away. Benchmark the ritual by showering with cool water before your next activity.

Farewell Mandala ✤ *Mandala de despedida*

This ritual is based on one I had never heard of until my father passed away in 2018, called *levantada de sombra* (lifting the shadow). My mother performed it beautifully in his honor. The objective is to lift the shadow, or spirit, of a deceased loved one to ensure that it moves forward into the next phase of existence. I envision this as the energy body moving into the energetic vastness or reuniting with Universal energy. In my research with family and friends, this ritual is considered the final farewell to a deceased loved one. It is performed for nine consecutive days after a death, the length of a novena in Catholicism. Most people in Mexico pass away in their homes, and it is typically performed on the physical ground where the loved one took their last breath. The original form of this ritual includes the use of candles and a large cross made of wood or flowers, which is why it is also sometimes called *levantada de cruz* (lifting of the cross).

The modern version of this ritual involves creating a mandala of flowers instead of a cross. A mandala is a geometric circular shape traditionally used as a visual meditation tool in Eastern philosophies. I find this shape and symbolism to be more inclusive than a cross, but the intention of the ritual does not vary. I suggest creating the mandala in the space of the deceased, if possible, and maintaining it for two to four days—or up to seven days if you are moved to do so.

Farewell Mandala Ritual

copalera

copal resin incense

incense charcoal and lighter

4–6 bunches of flowers

4–6 large bowls

10-inch dinner plate

spoon

1/4 cup pickling lime powder or Mexican cal (original mineral powder used)

5 candles

5 candleholders or small dishes

glass or vessel for water

cloth or shawl

photograph of the deceased

This ritual can be performed with the entire family. Depending on the intended size of the mandala, it can take a few hours. Begin by choosing the space for the mandala, lighting the incense in the copalera, and purifying the space with copal, leaving the incense lit throughout the process, if possible. Next, remove the flowers from the stems. Some flowers, such as roses or dahlias, can be used in full bloom; for others, such as chrysanthemums and carnations, you might choose to use just the petals. Place the petals and flowers in the bowls; you might want to separate them by color. Once you prepare the flowers, place the dinner plate at the center of the mandala site and, using the spoon, sprinkle the pickling lime or cal powder around the plate to the desired perimeter. Remove the plate, fill the circle with the powder, and place a candle at the center. Pickling lime is considered a purifying medium, and in this ritual, it helps to further cleanse the energy and absorb the shadow of the deceased.

Create the mandala by using the circle as a template, filling it with flowers and extending the circle until you reach a size you are happy with. You want to create a symmetrical shape that has some artistic expression; the stems can also be used artistically to create borders. Once this is done, place the four remaining candles in the candleholders in a square or diamond shape around the circle; these represent the four cardinal corners or directions. Adorn the candles as well with smaller circles of flowers. You can add more candles around the outer edges of the circle or integrate them into the center. You can also add smaller shapes on the outer edge of the circle to add more dimension. Place the glass of water and photograph at the North of the mandala or where the person's head would be located if you are creating this in the space of their passing. This is a contemplative practice; while you create this offering for your loved one, you can play soft music, chant mantras, pray, or offer a rosary if you are Catholic. The ritual is meant to open the heart while connecting to the deceased so that the emotion of grief can be expressed in a positive manner. The mandala will stay on the ground for two to four days; ideally, keep the candles lit the entire time.

Once the ritual feels complete, remove the flowers from the outside in and place them on the cloth. They can be taken to the cemetery and offered at the loved one's grave, composted, or offered back to Nature; what we don't want to do is keep them. The energy or vibration these flowers are meant to transmute should be released back to the Universe. This is the purpose of the ritual: to let go of the "shadow" so it moves on. Once the flowers are offered, it is customary to open the house to guests and hold a gathering, similar to a wake, in honor of the deceased. In Mexico, we offer Cacao and sweet bread to all of those who have participated in the ritual.

This beautiful ritual can be performed in the days or weeks following a funeral or cremation. It can also be part of a celebration of life or used to mark a remembrance day. The important part is to gather your family in gratitude and to express grief collectively, knowing you are not alone.

CHAPTER 8

VIBRACIÓN DEL CORAZÓN— ESSENCE OF THE HEART

The heart is the organ that keeps us alive by pumping blood through our entire body. It keeps its own particular rhythm. Medieval alchemists believed the heart was the location of the brain, while Buddhists have also proclaimed a heart-brain connection. The hypothesis is that when wisdom is truly integrated—not just learned—the decisions humans make are based on a compassionate, emotional state rather than an egotistical, logical state.

In curanderismo, the emotional heart is the key to healing. It is via the heart that the curandera/o can access the mind in a plática (chat). When one speaks truthfully from the heart, all misunderstandings, faults, and traumas are released and cleared. This is why many scholars of curanderismo consider it a form of psychotherapy. I recommend an excellent book by Antonio Noé

Zavaleta, PhD, *Curandero: Hispanic Ethno-Psychotherapy and Curanderismo* (2020), for a more clinical view on this subject. Whether the plática was influenced by the practice of religious confession during colonization, or arose from preserved Indigenous teachings, its use and emphasis is a cornerstone of curanderismo.

In this chapter, I will focus on the *emotional* heart. I firmly believe that while the brain is a logic center—where the mind can learn, envision, and process information—the heart is not only an emotional center but also the connection to Universal energy, the place where we build a connection to Spirit.

It is important to delineate how the emotional heart can affect us. From working with clients in private sessions, I have observed that a closed emotional heart can lead to *celos* (jealousy), *rabia* (rage), *melancolía* (depression), and *bilis* (acid reflux due to emotional outbursts), while an emotional heart that is too open can manifest as *mal de ojo* (evil eye), *adicción* (addiction), *egoísmo* (selfishness), and *ansiedad* (anxiety). Finding balance in the emotional heart is imperative for a harmonious life.

But how does one find balance? As emotional beings, we might experience these emotions at least once in our lives. Who hasn't felt celos over a neighbor's shiny new car? How many of us haven't had moments of ansiedad when faced with new and unknown life challenges? I find that a preventative approach through remedios y rituales supports us in finding the balance of the emotional heart. This means incorporating certain experiences or teachings into our lives as part of a daily, weekly, or monthly practice. Finding this routine will help us build resilience so that when emotions arise, we can face them and not let them overtake us.

REMEDIES—*REMEDIOS*

Cacao Elixir ✽ *Tónico de cacao*

Cacao (*L. Theobroma cacao*)—*Cacao*

ENERGY: Hot/dry | **TASTE:** Bitter and stimulating | **PLANT PART USED:** Seed/bean

Cacao has been a wonderful companion in my growth as a curandera. I attribute the grounding of my emotional heart to this plant ally. In 2015, I attended a women's Skillshare gathering called Spirit Weavers. I met an incredible Mexican woman named Paola who presented a cacao ceremony as part of her skill share. She was the first person to introduce me to cacao as an ancestral *medicina* (medicine) of the heart. From the first time I sat with her under the grandmother redwood trees in the forest of Northern California, cacao became a staple in my personal journey.

Before cacao, I had given no thought to offering one-on-one sessions. The idea of holding healing space for others was not a vision I held for my future. But slowly, as I sat weekly with cup after cup of cacao, I began to open up to sharing my gifts in a more personal and intimate manner. Cacao as a plant medicine opened my heart to a deeper understanding of service toward my community. I have since received teachings from Oaxacan and Guatemalan Maya lineages on cacao's ability to open communication, heart connections, and self-love, further expanding my heart to this plant's ability to heal us all.

Cacao is the plant from which chocolate is made. It is a flowering tree that bears oval, textured pods. Inside these pods are large seeds connected by a thick central vine that leads to the outside of the pod and connects to the branch. If you cut a cacao pod lengthwise, it resembles an ear of corn. In Guatemalan Mayan mythology, cacao and corn represent the duality of life. Cacao is the mother, and corn is the father; we, their children, cannot live without either. Cacao seeds have a white, sweet-tasting, fuzzy covering. Underneath, they are bitter and crunchy. These seeds undergo a process of fermentation, roasting, and peeling before they can be used. As a medicina, cacao is used in its unadulterated, raw state: *pasta de cacao* (cacao paste). The seeds are stone-ground into a thick paste for consumption. This process is still used in Mexico, Central America, and South America to make *chocolate caliente* (hot chocolate), a cacao drink made for special occasions, ceremonies, and community gatherings. An entire book could be dedicated to cacao, but for this introduction, we focus on its use as a ritualistic and heart-healing plant medicina. The recipes shared here are meant to bring harmony to your emotional heart.

Cacao's ability to nurture the metaphorical heart mirrors its physical action as a cardiovascular stimulant. In addition to being an antioxidant powerhouse, cacao contains essential minerals such as iron, potassium, and magnesium. Cacao also carries two important compounds—caffeine and theobromine—that act as vasodilators, dilating blood vessels and allowing blood to flow more smoothly. Blood flow promotes oxygenation of the body, leading to more energy, a calm mind, and an overall positive outlook.

Finding balance in the emotional heart means being aware of our own state of mind. As I have already mentioned, meditation and contemplative practices allow you to achieve this state through moments of quiet reflection. Before you begin any work with cacao, take some time to breathe deeply and find your center. Cacao is called Mama Cacao by the Maya and holds a special place in all the Americas as a sacred plant. Come to her in reverence, as a child to their mother, and she will soothe your heart.

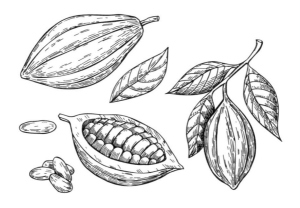

Cacao Elixir Recipe

1 cup water

1–4 tablespoons cacao paste, chopped

frother wand or 2 (8-ounce) cups (optional)

pinch of cinnamon powder

pinch of hot chili powder

preferred sweetener (optional)

In a small pot, bring the water to a boil; remove from the heat and add the cacao paste. Take your time melting the paste into the water, infusing it with your intentions as you mix it. When it is well-blended, add the sweetener, if desired, and use the frother wand for foaming. Alternatively, you can create foam by pouring the mixture repeatedly between two cups. Serve with a pinch of hot chili powder and cinnamon over the foam.

Suggested Use: Tónico de cacao can be served for personal rituals—after meditation, for example—or shared with your community or at small gatherings. The Maya in Guatemala serve a strong cup of cacao at their fire ceremonies, beginning with 1 tablespoon and working up to a maximum of 4 tablespoons. Keep in mind that cacao's high mineral content can lead to digestive imbalance and aggravate sensitivities to stimulants such as caffeine, so begin slowly and keep track of how you feel after drinking this tónico. Cacao's natural bitterness allows the plant's benefits to flow more easily through the body, as the bitter taste activates the liver. I encourage you to try the blend without sweetener; let it coat your tongue and sit in your stomach in its natural state. If you then feel called to add sugar, begin with small quantities.

Note on cacao for children: When I hold cacao circles and ceremonies, everyone is invited, including children. My rule of thumb is that if your child drinks coffee, they can partake in a small cup of cacao; if not, it might be better to skip it. For clarity, cacao is neither cocoa powder nor cacao powder; these powders are processed differently and may hold the flavor but not the espíritu or nutritional benefit of a cup of cacao made with cacao paste.

Rose Body Oil ❀ *Aceite corporal de rosas*

Rose (*L. Rosa centifolia*)—*Rosa*

ENERGY: Cold/Moist | PLANT PARTS USED: Flower petals

Geranium (*L. Pelargonium graveolens*)—*Geranio*

ENERGY: Cold | PLANT PARTS USED: Flower, leaf, and stem

Rosewood (*L. Aniba rosaeodora Ducke)—Palo de rosa*
ENERGY: Cold | **PLANT PART USED:** Buds

Frankincense (*L. Boswellia)—Franquincienso*
ENERGY: Hot/dry | **PLANT PARTS USED:** Resin

The rose is considered the queen of the plant world by many folk herbalists. It is the original emotional heart medicina introduced from Europe's schools of herbalism. I experienced this energy firsthand when I unintentionally poured an entire bottle of Bulgarian rose essential oil over my arm. The feeling of love bubbled up in me, along with a deep compassion for my fellow humans. I became aware of this shift in perception and began thinking back on the day's activities to discover what had changed—but the only difference in my routine was the rose essential oil accident. Since then, I have become a believer in its heart-opening benefits.

Today, rose is my number-one ally. I use it for personal self-care as well as recommend it and rely on it as a base in custom blends for my clients. It is beautiful to behold when rose medicina balances the emotional heart and allows for a true vibrational opening. Ayurveda places great emphasis on personal care as a ritual, and this particular body oil is inspired by Ayurvedic oils used for the self-care technique of abhyanga, a daily ritual that connects body and mind via massage.

As one of the most expensive essential oils on the planet, rose can be inaccessible to many. If necessary, it can be replaced with geranium leaf essential oil. The essential oils used in this body oil are complementary to each other; they offer heart opening and skin soothing benefits.

Abhyanga Body Oil Recipe

YIELD: approximately 16 ounces

1 cup rose petals

1 cup fractionated coconut oil

1 cup grapeseed or refined sesame oil, unscented

essential oils blend: 8 drops geranium leaf, 8 drops rosewood leaf, 6 drops frankincense, and 4–8 drops rose

1 (16-ounce) pump bottle

Pulverize the rose petals in a blender. Infuse them into the coconut oil following the instructions for Oil Infusion (page 35), using the double-boiler method for a 2-hour infusion. Strain and return the infused oil to the double boiler, adding the grapeseed oil. Stir until the mixture is fully incorporated. Remove it from the heat, let it cool for 10 minutes, and add the essential oils blend; mix well and let cool. Transfer the rose body oil to the pump bottle, cover tightly, and store in a cool, dark place.

Suggested Use: Abhyanga as a ritual requires time and intention. Although Ayurvedic instruction suggests oiling and massaging every day, I recommend two to three times a week. If this strains your schedule, begin with once a week. This practice can bring balance to the emotional heart by helping you connect to your body. It is an excellent ritual for anyone who suffers from physical abuse trauma, a closed heart, or a frigid disposition.

In preparation for the ritual, you will need a towel, a small pot with water, a small (1-pint) mason jar, access to a heat source, and the rose body oil. Add sufficient body oil to the mason jar to spread on your entire body. Place the jar in the pot with water, in a bain-marie, warming the oil to a comfortable temperature.

Sitting on the towel, begin massaging toward the heart—up from the feet, in from the hands, and finally down from the scalp. As you massage, keep a visual in your mind's eye of a soft pink light at the heart. You can recite a loving affirmation such as "I am love, I am worthy, I am complete" as you massage. Play music if that feels intuitive. This ritual will leave you feeling simultaneously lighter in the heart and grounded, as somatic practices tend to do. In Ayurvedic tradition, this massage is performed before washing the body with water. Aside from the touch benefit, oiling the body in this manner can help retain moisture and keep the skin soft.

Rose, Cacao, and Hibiscus Devotional Syrup ❁ *Jarabe de rosas, cacao, y flor de Jamaica para uso de devoción*

ENERGY: Cooling/dry then hot/dry | TASTE: Sweet/sour

This recipe incorporates rose and cacao for a sweet and flavorful devotional infusion. The hibiscus lends a beautiful color and crowns this blend with an added tart flavor. When making sacred preparaciónes, it is important to add a sweet note. Making this syrup with a glycerin base makes it easy on the tongue and does not interfere with your devotional practices. Sweetness is a naturally comforting taste; unlike bitter or pungent tastes, sweet tastes call upon the energy of attraction.

This blend will ground your physical energy with roasted cacao peel, while its natural caffeine will keep your body energized. The rose petals in this formula will promote emotional heart activation and expand the energy of love and devotion, while the hibiscus will brighten the tongue with tartness and kindle the liver to assimilate the benefits of the formula.

Devotional Syrup Recipe

YIELD: approximately 32 ounces

2 ounces roasted cacao peel

3 ounces rose petals

1 ounce hibiscus, cut and sifted

8 ounces water

32-ounce mason jars with lid

24 ounces glycerin

cloth sieve

dropper bottles

Prepare the cacao peel, rose petals, and hibiscus by briefly pulsing them in a blender—not pulverizing them, but breaking up the surface areas for better infusion. Boil the water and mix it with the herb mixture in a mason jar; steep for 30 minutes. Add the glycerin, cover, and shake lightly. Store in a cool, dark place for two to four weeks, checking the flavor at week 2 and decanting by week 4. Strain the infusion through the cloth sieve into a clean mason jar for storing, squeezing the hierbas to extract maximum flavor and color. Dispense into dropper bottles for serving.

Suggested Use: Take one full dropper under the tongue before your devotional, meditation, or contemplative practices. Ingesting this devotional syrup will help bring awareness to the emotional heart. It can also be diluted by adding two droppers to 1 cup of warm water or milk. This comforting formula is also a good choice for moving through grief and deep emotional releases.

RITUALS—*RITUALES*

Rose Petal Bath and Ritual ✿
Baño y ritual de rosas

This baño is different from the Basin Herb Bath (page 69). Roses are its singular ingredient. This is a modern version of a *barrida de rosas* (rose sweep), a traditional curanderismo ritual for alleviating heartbreak, grief, and depression. It is also similar to a ritual described by Elena Avila in *Woman Who Glows in the Dark* (2000), which treats trauma through mock burial. I had never heard of this and was surprised both to know it existed and to realize I had tapped into ancestral knowledge.

My love of rose inspired this ritual. I first envisioned it for a client who had experienced a deep loss. If you are open to experimenting with this ritual for yourself, I suggest you find a confidante who can help you through the process, although I will suggest some ways to do it on your own.

2 dozen roses	small bowl
basin or large pot	ritual water
1 cup rose hydrosol or rose water	queen-size cotton blanket
	1–2 pillows

Put one rose aside; prepare the rest of the flowers by removing all of the petals and placing them in the basin or pot. Add ¼ cup of the rose hydrosol or rose water to dampen the petals but not completely saturate them. As you do this, focus on your breath. Remain quiet and contemplate the healing work you want to ask of

Hermana Rosa (Sister Rose). Place the remaining liquid in the small bowl with a splash of ritual water; lay the single rose on the side. Prepare your body by showering.

Lie on the blanket next to the basin or pot and adjust the pillow(s) for comfort.

Take a couple of deep breaths, focusing on the expansion of the chest and heart on the inhale and releasing completely on the exhale. When you feel your mind clearing, cover yourself with the rose petal–rose water mixture, beginning at your feet and working up to your head. Either on your own or with assistance, wrap yourself loosely with the blanket, and when you are completely covered, breathe and focus on your heart center. Allow for emotions to emerge. This will manifest in different ways for everyone. Let tears and words exit your body, but take care not to yell or thrash about, as Hermana Rosa embodies gentle energy. I encourage you to both release your emotions and stay present to them. It is in this conscious presence that you will find breakthroughs and real empowerment for healing.

When finished, unwrap your body and remove the rose petals. Use the set-aside rose water to lightly wash your physical body and close the energy of the vibrational body. When ready, rise and wrap the rose petals in the blanket to discard later. Take some time to rest and hydrate your body. This ritual can be beautifully performed outdoors in a shaded area where you will be undisturbed for 15–30 minutes.

If you have access to a bathtub, this ritual can be performed in the same way and without assistance. In this scenario, you can dispense with the blanket. The ideal position for this ritual is to lie in the fetal position.

Suggested Use: This is a rejuvenating ritual for those going through grieving or for anyone who needs to bring balance to their emotional heart. It can be performed once a month for three months to restore harmony.

CHAPTER 9

ESPÍRITU DE LAS FLORES—ESSENCE OF THE FLOWERS

This chapter is special to me—it is an opportunity to share all I have learned about vibrational healing and wellness. Espíritu de las flores refers to the power of flower essences. I translate this use of *espíritu* as "essence" rather than "spirit," as the latter word is laden with too many indoctrinated, religious definitions that carry heavy energy, in my opinion. "Essence" speaks to the abstract nature of the word.

Having now read the previous chapters, there is much to unlearn, because when we talk about the vibrational or energetic body, we no longer use the same approach to healing. The hierbas used in the remedios presented thus far have largely been for physical ailments. In curanderismo and Latine herbalism, the material constituents and botanical actions influence the physical body very concretely. The use of hierbas in rituales is symbolic and intuitive—sometimes they are chosen for superstitious reasons; it might depend on whether the practitioner is a Latine folk herbalist or a curandera/o. As a teacher of curanderismo, my personal pursuit has been to define and provide more structure around the hierbas and flores we choose for rituales, in order to teach more practically and cohesively.

In my curanderismo practice, I find the use of rituales to be the link that switches the brain from doing to being. Rituales move us out of the "thinking mind" into a "believing mind," revealing our connection to Universal energy. They feed our need for presence and devotion and allow for the creative part of the mind to open. When performed consistently, they can become a form of meditation or contemplative practice, briefly quieting the "thinking mind."

In this chapter, I want to empower you to build your own rituales with confidence. We have already covered the two basic rituales in curanderismo: the limpias or barridas (energy cleanses or sweeps) and baños (baths). If you agree that it would be useful for you to pick your own hierbas and flores for these rituales without following a recipe, know that you *can* work intuitively—but intuition, as I learned from one of my meditation teachers, is built from active experience. I hope to share some interesting information on hierbas and flores that will inspire you to test and enjoy creating your own formulas. Hopefully, along the way, you can also gain the necessary experience to access and trust your intuition.

We will begin at the beginning, when symbolism and attributes beyond the physical were given to the plant world. The doctrine of signatures (DOS) originates from Roman-Greek botany and was used extensively in alchemical and Hermetic traditions, which sought to understand how the macrocosm (universe) corresponds to the microcosm (individual). DOS believed that the shape, color, and growing patterns of a plant correlated to the shape, color, and patterns of diseases and ailments. For example, beans resemble kidneys; therefore, their signature, or vibrational alignment, was to the kidney organs, and the remedy for kidney stones was to eat lots of beans! As you can imagine, these remedies might not have been entirely reliable, but writings as late as the seventeenth century praise this healing methodology. If you are interested in a modern take on DOS, Julia Graves's book *The Language of Plants: A Guide to the Doctrine of Signatures* (2012) is a must-read. Julia was one of my first teachers in folk herbalism and flower essences. Her inclusive teachings gave me confidence and inspired me to share curanderismo more broadly. Unlike herbalism, which uses the phrase "modality of opposites," the doctrine of signatures is a "modality of similars"; as the bean example illustrates, the ailment and remedy are in alignment—in this case, the shapes align. Although we no longer use DOS for its herbalism teachings, it forms the foundation of my teachings on vibrational or energetic healing; the hierbas and flores we choose are based on the modality of similars.

Many of curanderismo's remedios y rituales address the results of unbalanced emotional states, such as susto (shock), mal de ojo (evil eye), and melancolía (depression). The emotional and mental state of a person reveals whether the vibrational or energetic body has suffered an injury. Because we cannot see it, we rely on our perception of mental and emotional states. When someone experiences a surprising life event or traumatic experience, their attitude and way of thinking are altered—even when there is no change to their physical body or day-to-day life.

Duelo (grief) exemplifies this; it generally occurs when someone we love passes away, and while we don't experience a physical assault, the emotional feeling of deep sadness can result in fatigue, apathy, or depression. This should not be equated with any physical chemical changes that stem from birth, such as autism or chemical depression. It is important to keep this in mind, as sometimes we need herbal preparations or a limpia, and sometimes we need medication. Knowing the difference means having self-awareness of who we are, how we react to life experiences, and what makes us feel whole and complete.

THE BASICS OF VIBRATIONAL REMEDIOS

In chapter 2, I shared some basic information about the vibrational body. Here, we will go into more depth. I like to teach that the vibrational body might not be seen, but it can be felt and perceived. The studies of Dr. Joe Dispenza have shown us that a perceivable shift in electromagnetic waves occurs when a person meditates. In scientific terms, an electromagnetic wave is energy, and energy is everywhere, emanating from both animate and inanimate objects.

The energy of electromagnetic waves can be perceived in thermal, visual, and auditory ways. Thermal energy is perceived from heat—the sun being the largest example. Visual energy is perceived from light and color; for instance, the colors of a rainbow are reflections of light in water particles, and the color of a flower is the reflection of light through solid particles. Auditory energy includes radio waves that have been developed into TV, Wi-Fi, and Bluetooth. Energy surrounds us, and we have become experts in manipulating it.

For our purposes, we are focused on visual energy, the energy of color and light. The color spectrum measured in wavelengths tells us that darker colors have long wavelengths, while lighter colors have short wavelengths. More specifically, when we refer to wavelengths, we mean how the particles move at a microscopic level. Denser particles move slowly—their wavelengths are longer, hence "heavier." Less condensed particles move faster with shorter wavelengths, making them "lighter." We can relate darker colors to heavier energy and lighter colors to lighter energy.

My personal concept of vibrational healing developed over the past decade through extensive observation. I grew to understand that a flower's color vibration needed to be in resonance with the ailment it was addressing, and that a resonance of similarity, like the doctrine of signatures, was key to achieving healing. When two elements are on the same wavelength, a positive attraction of energy results. In contrast, opposing wavelengths result in neutrality. Sound healing duplicates this finding; musical notes that are in alignment, or resonance, create a sense of comfort and relief, while notes that are not in alignment create dissonance.

Although I am not the first to delve into this concept, I use it to explain how energy healing works. If you have ever used Bach flower remedies, the underlying concept is the same. Flower essences are vibrational remedies; they are not essential oils or distillations. The energy of a flower is imprinted into water, and this water is used for healing support. A similarity must exist between the flower and the ailment for the essence to produce results. My favorite example is the bleeding heart flower essence. I use this flower to treat heartbreak and grief because it resembles a heart cut in half. Instead of using a cheerful daylily to attempt to restore the energy of joy to a grieving person, healing is accomplished through the resonance of the person's energy that matches a flower that looks like a bleeding heart cut in half. Vibrational or energetic healing occurs on a subtle, nuanced level. I share this approach as a tool for your self-healing journey. I also encourage you to test it for yourself.

ORGANIZING VIBRATIONAL HEALING

Now that we have some basic information, I can offer more details on common ailments and the hierbas, flores, and *elementos* (elements) needed for optimal wellness support in vibrational energetic healing. The ailment dictates whether a vibrational remedy or a ritual is called for. At times, it is difficult to separate the ritual from the remedy. This is where intuition and experience are valuable. The one component that can never be lacking is the plática. If you are practicing self-care and self-healing, the plática can be integrated into your treatment by keeping a journal for self-analysis, allowing you to review your mental and emotional state along the way. If you are sharing your gifts with someone, it requires holding yourself and them accountable for their progress with weekly pláticas. This is the space in which you will notice signs of healing and assess the effectiveness of the vibrational remedios y rituales.

Shape

Flowers are the pinnacle and purpose of a plant. I describe them as the uteri of plants—it is from this space that a plant reproduces and bears fruit that carries the seed, initiating a new cycle of plants. Because of this crucial role, flowers hold enormous power and a high level of vibrational energy. They have traditionally occupied an exalted place in curanderismo.

Shape and color determine a flower's use in vibrational healing. Its shape may resonate with an organ, or its color with an ailment's energy. Or, a person can resonate with a particular flower. I personally resonate with the rose family of flowers, which expands my ability to use roses for healing purposes. The layer-upon-layer arrangement of rose petals resonates with the multiple layers of the vibrational body, and the petal shape itself aligns with the shape of the heart. For more details on flower shape, I recommend Julia's book, which contains extensive information based on the doctrine of signatures. Experiment with several flowers until you find one that speaks to you clearly and assists you in healing.

Color

I find that the flower's shape or symbolism is less important than its color. Through observation and experimentation, I have made some connections between flower color and vibrational qualities. Chart E will provide some shortcuts, but take some time to tune into the vibrational qualities for yourself.

Chart E: The Tissue States in TWH and Curanderismo/Latine Herbalism

COLOR	VIBRATIONAL QUALITIES/ENERGY RESONANCE
Black, brown	Neutralizes the energy of physical trauma; grounding energy similar to the Earth element; resonates with temperance, lack of energy, inertia, stagnation, heaviness, lethargy
Red, purple	Slightly stimulating energy; resonates with rejuvenation, firmness, overthinking, inertia, grief, fear, melancholy
Magenta, pink	Cooling and bright energy; resonates with happiness, connection, anxiety, stress, worry, nervousness
Orange	Warm and stimulating energy; resonates with expansion, creativity, manifestation, joy, overstimulation, overwhelm, desire
Yellow	Stimulating energy similar to the Fire element; resonates with clearing, transformation, aggression, transition, anger
Green	Calming energy; resonates with restraint, relaxation, lethargy
Indigo, blue	Restful energy similar to the Water element; resonates with moderation, sleep, understimulation, sedation, sadness, tension
Violet	Cooling energy similar to the Air element; resonates with sadness, low mental process, frigidity, tension
White	Neutralizes the energy of emotional trauma; resonates with protection, purity, shock, surprise

HERBS AND FLOWERS— *HIERBAS Y FLORES*

I have observed a common thread regarding hierbas and flores among curanderas/os in Mexico, Guatemala, Nicaragua, and Cuba in their reliance on the modality of similars. Generally, any bitter hierba can be used for a limpia, as its astringent properties "cut through" any unwanted vibrations. Hot hierbas are used for stimulating vibrational energy, as the warming properties can stimulate blood flow. Cold hierbas are used for grounding and relaxing vibrations, as the cooling properties are used to "tonify" the nervous system; specific examples are provided in Chart F on page 132. When we make herbal preparations with the correct hierbas, the physical healing is immediately apparent. Likewise, when we

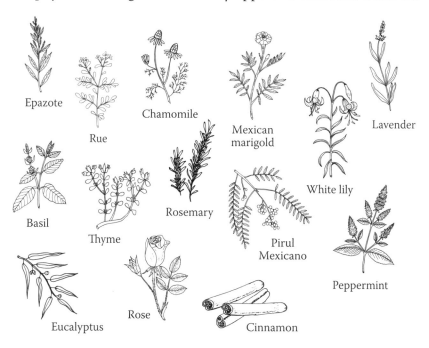

Epazote

Rue

Chamomile

Mexican marigold

Lavender

Basil

Thyme

Rosemary

White lily

Pirul Mexicano

Peppermint

Eucalyptus

Rose

Cinnamon

prepare vibrational remedies with their resonating elements, the energetic results are felt even before we administer them. After all, energy is not bound by physical constraints.

Chart F: Physical Qualities, Vibrational Resonance, and Corresponding Herbs

HERB PHYSICAL QUALITY	HERB VIBRATIONAL RESONANCE
Bitter	Neutralizing energy; resonates with clearing, protection, inertia, stagnation, heaviness, overthinking, worry, shock EXAMPLES: Chamomile, *epazote* (Mexican wormseed), *ruda* (rue)
Hot	Energizing and stimulating energy; resonates with clearing, rejuvenation, fear, anxiety, nervousness, overstimulation, overwhelm, aggression, anger EXAMPLES: Cinnamon, thyme, rosemary, basil, epazote, ruda, *Pirul Mexicano* (*L. Schinus molle*; Mexican pepper tree), *cempasúchil* (Mexican marigold)
Cold	Grounding and relaxing energy; resonates with protection, melancholy, grief, sadness, tension, frigidity EXAMPLES: Chamomile, *menta* (mint), eucalyptus, rose, lilies, lavender

ELEMENTS

Chart G on page 133 provides an abbreviated version of the elemental qualities for vibrational healing. Keep these in mind when formulating your rituals. It is always beneficial to invoke the energy of an element in your rituals for a deeper connection.

Chart G: Vibrational Qualities of Elements

ELEMENT	VIBRATIONAL QUALITY
Earth	Heavy; dense, slow-moving
	EXAMPLES: Crystals, flowers, plants
Fire	Dense; hot, stimulating, transformative
	EXAMPLES: Candles, ritual fire
Water	Fluid; degrees of stimulation range from flow (flowing water) to inertia (frozen water)
	EXAMPLES: Floral water, ritual water, holy water
Air	Flux; degrees of stimulation range from swirl (breeze) to overstimulating (tornado)
	EXAMPLES: Incense, smudging, feathers
Ether	Resonates directly with the vibrational body; resonance with Universal energy
	EXAMPLES: Devotional images and statues

AILMENTS

In many places in the Americas, curanderas/os are called upon for their expertise in vibrational healing. Following is a list of ailments commonly treated in curanderismo that I can share from a place of certainty. The resonating vibrational qualities that can support healing are also listed. Use the corresponding flower color chart (Chart E) and herb resonance chart (Chart F) to locate the appropriate hierbas and flores for your rituals.

Note: These are not clinical terms; the definitions originate from my interactions and observations with clients over time.

Abuso sexual (sexual abuse): Unwanted sexual interaction of any kind—especially at a young age, where child-adult boundaries are crossed

Corresponding Vibrational Energy: Neutralizing, protective, grounding, calming

Adicción (addiction): Physical response to abuse, overstimulation, grief, depression, worry, or anger

Corresponding Vibrational Energy: Transformative, grounding

Ansiedad (anxiety): Overstimulation of the mind that is so severe it begins to develop into physical attacks, pain, and/or complete inertia

Corresponding Vibrational Energy: Grounding, calming

Bilis (acid reflux due to emotional outbursts): Mostly affects children and teens; digestive issues due to tantrums

Corresponding Vibrational Energy: Grounding, neutralizing, purifying

Celos y envidia (jealousy and envy): Giving overstimulating energy to others

Corresponding Vibrational Energy: Neutralizing, transformative

Depresión (depression): Deep, accumulated grief that can lead to thoughts of suicide

Corresponding Vibrational Energy: Neutralizing, protective

Duelo (grief): Heavy sadness over the loss of someone or something loved so deeply that life becomes unbearable

Corresponding Vibrational Energy: Stimulating, transformative, purifying, grounding

Egoísmo (**selfishness**): Lack of sympathy, mental response to lack of enrichment, or the result of overprotection

Corresponding Vibrational Energy: Neutralizing, grounding

Enojo (**unprovoked anger**): Internal mental stimulation stemming from unhappiness, silenced opinions, or unrequited love

Corresponding Vibrational Energy: Neutralizing, calming, grounding

Frialdad (**frigidity**): Lack of interest in mental stimulation manifesting as unemotional; lack of interest in sexual touch or interaction; severe shyness

Corresponding Vibrational Energy: Stimulating, calming, grounding

Mal de ojo (**evil eye**): Receiving overstimulating energy from others

Corresponding Vibrational Energy: Neutralizing, purifying, protective

Melancolía (**melancholy**): Lack of interest in life due to overstimulation or overprotection

Corresponding Vibrational Energy: Stimulating, grounding

Obsesión (**obsession**): Mental response to desire, unrequited love, jealousy, or overstimulation, overprotection

Corresponding Vibrational Energy: Transformative, calming, grounding

Preocupación (**worry**): Overthinking with a negative focus

Corresponding Vibrational Energy: Grounding, calming

Rabia (**rage**): Emotional outbursts due to compounded fear and unhappiness

Corresponding Vibrational Energy: Purifying, neutralizing, calming, grounding

Resentimiento (**resentment**): Resulting from grief, anger, or lack of nurturing

Corresponding Vibrational Energy: Transformative, grounding

Separación de relaciones (**separation or divorce**): Broken heart, unrequited love, releasing emotional relationships to move forward in life

Corresponding Vibrational Energy: Transformative, grounding, stimulating

Susto (**shock or PTSD**): Mental trauma stemming from verbal abuse, physical abuse, or unexpected or tragic news and revelations

Corresponding Vibrational Energy: Neutralizing, grounding, purifying, calming

FLOWER ESSENCES

Flower essences are my favorite remedio for supporting vibrational wellness. They are traditionally ingested but can also be applied topically. They are usually administered for specific periods— long-term or short-term—depending on the ailment that needs to be rebalanced. Consistent use supports the repatterning of vibrational body energies. As I share in my Reiki circles and cacao ceremonies, physical changes can affect the vibrational body, and reciprocally, vibrational changes can affect the physical body.

Flower essences are the bottled vibrational energy of flowers and are safe to use. They can be added to baths, applied to acupressure points, and misted over the body. Children, animals, and anyone, whether healthy or frail, can receive the benefits of flower essences, as they are subtle and easy to use.

The focus in using vibrational remedios is to support your vibrational body and mental-emotional state. I recommend building a small library, starting with two or three remedies that you can experience before you begin to share this treatment with others. I experimented for six years before using flower essences in my practice to ensure that I understood somatically how these remedios worked—not just theoretically or from a book. Working with a vibrational healer can also be invaluable.

I make my own flower essences from flowers grown in my garden for this specific purpose, with roses being my personal favorite. Making these essences is an advanced skill, and with the availability of quality manufacturers, it is not entirely necessary. But learning how to use them, along with the basic terminology, is essential.

There are three degrees of flower essences:

- **Mother:** original, undiluted vibrational essence. It is kept in a sun-free environment, separated from other remedies, especially essential oils, and away from radio waves and electronics. It is rarely used as a remedy itself. Mothers are deeply transformational; dilution is necessary to avoid causing mental or emotional imbalance. Remember, flower essences are pure energy, and excess energy disturbs and causes dissonance.

- **Stock:** mother essence once diluted. This second-degree vibrational remedio is sometimes available for purchase.
- **Dose:** stock essence, further diluted. This third-degree vibrational remedio is the form that is traditionally available for purchase.

Dosing guidelines are as follows:
- **Stock-degree flower essence:** 1 drop under the tongue or 1 drop three to four times a day.
- **Dose-degree flower essence:** 3–4 drops under the tongue three to four times a day. If this frequency is unmanageable, you can add the full dose of 9–16 drops to a water bottle and drink it throughout the day.
- **For use on the body:** Apply 1 drop of stock-degree flower essence or 2 drops of dose-degree, up to three times a day.
- **For use in a mister:** Mix 1 part brandy and 3 parts spring water in a 2-ounce spray bottle, adding up to 6 drops of dose-degree flower essence. Spray face and head two to three times a day to alleviate discomfort or whenever you feel the need.
- **For use in a limpia:** Add up to 4 drops of dose-degree flower essence directly to the fresh herbs.
- **For use in a baño:** Add 2–3 drops of dose-degree flower essence along with the flowers.

I have studied with some European makers of flower essences who specify highly detailed uses for flower essences, but I find that the method Julia introduced me to is more intuitive and effective.

To discontinue the use of flower essences or vibrational remedios, one can either consciously move away from consistent use, forgetting or no longer feeling called to use them, or work one-on-one with a healer until the treatment results in a mental or emotional change.

I suggest the following flower essences as a beginner's repertoire.

- **Red rose:** aligns with denser qualities and emotions
- **Pink yarrow:** serves as a protective energy shield
- **Magenta bougainvillea:** aligns with dense energy and sharp emotions
- **Orange cempasúchil:** resonates with stimulating energy of the vibrational body
- **Yellow dahlia:** connects to the solar energy in the body
- **Violet orchid:** softens the energy of the mind and emotions
- **White rose:** calls on the energy of purity

VIBRATIONAL HEALING

In curanderismo, vibrational healing derives from limpias and baños. In addition to using sweeping actions, limpias also provide direct contact with the body through tapping and rubbing the skin with the chosen hierbas and flores. Baños use water as a vehicle. In the traditions of the Amazon tribes and the Maya in Guatemala, I have seen how they use baños in a time-honored fashion. Baños are done in community in large vats and require huge quantities of herbs. The herbs are boiled, releasing the aromatics, and special ritual waters are added before scrubbing the entire body with the hot mixture. In Mexican and Cuban curanderismo, the basin baño is smaller and more contained but yields the same result. One commonality between these traditions is the use of limpias to liberate stagnant, heavy energies and using baños for protection or the release of deep trauma.

Choosing Vibrational Remedios

You now have information about vibrational healing and can confidently choose supportive remedios for your needs. Here is a simple list to help you move through this process with ease.

Ailment: _____

Hierbas: _____

Flower color: _____

Flower essences: _____

Supportive element: _____

Type of remedio: limpia/baño

Date and time of remedio: _____

Mental, emotional state before remedio: _____

_____

_____

_____

Mental, emotional state after remedio: _____

_____

_____

_____

Integration and reflection: _____

_____

_____

_____

Other support as necessary: _____

_____

_____

For a limpia, I recommend choosing one herb and one flower; for a baño, one herb and two flowers. Alternatively, only hierbas or only flores can be used. When working with energy, less is more. A focused approach to healing will always deliver the clearest results. Use an intuitive approach when pairing remedios with ailments—I often ask my students to choose their remedios first, then we work in reverse to determine the ailment. This is an interesting experiment that has led many students to become aware of hidden energy dissonance.

Remember to choose your hierbas and flores from organic sources if you are unable to grow your own. For limpias, always use fresh hierbas and flores to make your bouquets. You can enhance their healing properties by placing them on your altar or in your sacred space one day before use. Fresh or dried herbs are acceptable for baños, but flowers should be fresh, if possible, as these call on the energies of richness and life abundance. I recommend that beginners choose one manufacturer among the many brands of flower essences and learn their repertoire. This will give you a notion of the range of possibilities offered.

Sacred Space

The place where you perform your rituales needs to be private, safe, and sacred. It can be in your garden, hidden from neighbors' eyes, in a separate room in your home, or even in a yurt, as mine is.

Organizing your sacred space is principally about finding a comfortable place that can contain the energy as you practice rituals. First, establish a place for a stationary altar. Altars are the portals that connect us to the matrix of Universal energy, and this connection should be nurtured and honored. Altars are also sites for grieving, praying, and reflecting our devotion. I have a stationary altar in my home and a mobile altar I use when making house calls, traveling, and practicing in the yurt. The altar can be simple, with four symbolic items connecting to the four elements of earth, fire, water, and air, and one item connecting the altar to your devotional belief. As you become more experienced, you will naturally want to add more items to this portal of energy that resonate with your essence.

Moreover, an altar is an extension of a practitioner's energy. Elena Avila shares in *Woman Who Glows in the Dark* (2000) that the first thing she did with her clients before beginning her rituals and healing work was to introduce them to her altar. It became an entity unto itself. Another example of the importance of altars is the Shrine Room in the Rubin Museum of Art in

NYC, which housed a number of Buddhist altars for years before recently transferring to the Brooklyn Museum of Art. Vibrational shifts are known to occur in people just by sitting in the presence of these altars. For any serious practitioner of curanderismo, an altar in your sacred space is mandatory.

Your sacred space should be uncluttered and neat to support open and unfettered thought and communication. Cleanliness allows for the energy to flow. This space will become a place of personal reflection and, in time, emotional release. It will eventually be where you practice your rituals, express your devotion, build the vibration of your practice, and discover your personal style of healing.

CONCLUSION: FINDING YOUR PRACTICE

As a Mexican-Cuban-American woman, it has taken me years to learn about my mixed heritage, and I am still uncovering spaces that need love and attention. I am forever grateful to be able to share my personal story and knowledge with you. I hope this book will support you in finding *your* practice. The hierbas, remedios, and rituales discussed here are just the beginning of reclaiming Latine culture. Reach out to your family members; I know they will have knowledge to expand on what is shared here. My ultimate wish for you is that you uncover your family heritage and forge a deeper connection to your ancestors. If this book has served as even a spark for a conversation about your grandmother's tea, it would please me to know you are diving deeper into your *latinidad* (Latine culture). *¡Hasta luego!*

CURANDERISMO: A LIVING TRADITION THROUGH INTERVIEWS

It gives me great pleasure to introduce you, dear reader, to a few curanderas/os who hold unique points of view. As soon as I met these wonderful people, I knew they carried the living traditions of curanderismo in their blood. They inspire me with their personal practices and their devotion to the restoration and decolonization of the ancestral ways of healing. You will find that their words parallel some of what I have shared in this book and, in some cases, offer new paths for inspiration.

YAYA ERIN RIVERA

I met Yaya in 2015 at a women's Skillshare gathering called Spirit Weavers. We had an inexplicable connection from the beginning. She was one of the first people who spoke about plants and energy in the same way I did. Later on, we came to see that our Taíno ancestry—hers from Borikén (Puerto Rico) and mine from Cuba—must have recognized itself through our DNA. I hold a special place in my heart for Yaya; she inspires me with her openness, "weirdness" (a very good thing in our community!), and incredibly large heart. I hope you find in her words a path to relearning the ancestral ways. She carries the medicina (medicine) of recolonization and integration.

What is your full name? Include title (if you have one) and whether it is a self- or community-given title.

My name is Yaya Erin Rivera, and I am a Folk Medicine Practitioner. As a mixed person, I chose this title because it is general enough to include both my Irish Celtic ancestry, in which many of my activities fall under the title of Druid, and my Taíno lineage, in which I might be called a curandera or *bruja* (witch), depending on the lens that my life is being viewed through. I feel that this title, being in English, also acknowledges my upbringing in the United States, where destiny first revealed to me a path as a Green Witch and herbalist in the Wise Woman Tradition. Although being the first generation in my motherline to be born in the United States has been painful and confusing to navigate, it has also given me the privilege of studying many different approaches to plants and personal and planetary health. For me, this language makes room for all of those realities to harmoniously coexist.

Where were you born, and where is your Latine heritage from?

I was born in Connecticut, of all places! As far back as we have records, my motherline is from the island of Borikén. My mother, Migdalia; grandmother, Rafaela; great-grandmother, Leonarda; and great-great-grandmother, Santiaga, to my knowledge, were all born in Cayey, Puerto Rico.

Can you share a little about your journey into the healing arts?

Like many Taínos, my ancestors endured a lot of hardships due to colonization and genocide, and I feel my motherline is still recovering from the individualistic, extractive values of the colonizing culture. This shows up as hereditary chronic illness, and my mother, grandmother, and I were all diagnosed with a variety of chronic illnesses that hormonal fluctuations at puberty and menopause exacerbated greatly. Western doctors had no idea what to make of my symptoms, and I started seeing energy workers, doing lymphatic body rolling, and experimenting with medical diets and herbal tinctures at the age of sixteen, when most of my peers were focused on emotional and social growth, grades, and partying. My mother became a yoga teacher around that time, and we did a lot of exploring of visual and healing arts modalities together. While in art school in New York City, I devoured every opportunity to heal that came my way, visiting many different kinds of healers in quest of a working under-standing of how to be a good steward of the body I was given. In some ways, I felt my teen and young adult years were taken from me, and in retrospect, I can see that I didn't come to this life just for a vacation; I got started on my true calling and its curriculum early on. I drank ayahuasca for the first time in a fancy yoga studio in Manhattan. In that space, I was guided to leave New York City and move to an Earthship in New Mexico to give birth to my son. I have a special relationship with underpopulated/wild places and often go into a type of hermitage to incubate big changes in my life, grow, and give birth to the next version of myself.

How do you define Latine herbalism, and when were you introduced to it?

The first memory I have of a homemade herbal remedy is my Nana Rafaela going out to her backyard garden in suburban Connecticut, picking fresh rue, stuffing it in a plastic bottle of isopropyl rubbing alcohol from the drugstore, and using it as a liniment for leg cramps at night. Knowing the plants and how to care for daily aches and pains, cuts, and scrapes at home was not considered specialty knowledge like it is in the States today. This was just part of being a woman, being a mother, and caring for your family. On a family visit to Puerto Rico when I was maybe fourteen, I found María Benedetti's book *Earth and Spirit: Medicinal Plants and Healing Lore from Puerto Rico* (1989) and read about elders openly sharing our traditional Puerto Rican ways of healing for the first time in ways that felt exciting. Growing up, the gifts of intuition and healing that run in our family were still labeled as "devil worship," and I was cautioned and pressured by many to hide that side of myself. Instead, owing to my rebellious spirit, I became a rural teenage pagan and read every book on magic and healing I could get my hands on in the small mom-and-pop bookshops of the neighboring towns.

I initiated as a Green Witch in my twenties and worked with the plants common to the land where I lived as a Wise Woman herbalist for around eight years, integrating what I had been taught into my way of life.

All the while, I longed for elders of my maternal lineage to really study and go deep with. It took many years of searching before I found Alfonso Peralta (www.tainostudies.org) and Akutu Irka Mateo of Sacred Taíno Healing to share language, cultural context, cosmovision, and remedies in the way I had been seeking. The Wise Woman tradition teaches us to access and be nourished by the accumulated wisdom of our own ancestors. I honor that lineage as a foundation that gave me a working knowledge of the plants around me so I could begin to heal my body enough to put forth the effort required to dig deeper and do the necessary decolonization, unearthing, and reclaiming of what for many generations had been considered lost in my heritage. Until fairly recently, the common belief was that the Taíno were extinct; but we are still here, in community, finding each other and finding the safety to allow ourselves to be seen, to raise our voices, and say, "We're still here!" I see Latine herbalism as another way of talking about the forms of traditional Afro-Caribbean folk medicine that survived colonization. I feel that, in these times, we are called to the important work of picking up and weaving back together all the pieces of our good, Earth-honoring traditions that colonizing forces attempted to destroy and integrating them into a good way of walking that is right for these times.

Do you have a personal relationship with curanderismo?

I do not. We use the term "curandera" for healer in a general way in some Taíno spiritual communities I am part of, but I am aware that there is a different culture around the concept of curanderismo in Mexico, which I have not been formally initiated into. My studies have leaned more toward Amazonian plant medicine and nutrition, as the Taíno came originally from the Andes down the Orinoco River in canoes and made their way to various Caribbean islands, like Puerto Rico, Haiti, the Dominican Republic, Cuba, Jamaica, and the Virgin Islands. I find that many Amazonian tribes still eat the traditional foods of my Taíno ancestors and work with some of our known medicinal plants, and so I feel compelled to go as far back as I can to understand the big picture of who and how my people have been, and how that influences the personal and collective challenges we face today. I can identify as Latine, but my path with plants has been more through Arawak culture, food, music, and medicines like cacao, tobacco, and psilocybin. These studies coexist within me alongside the Indigenous-European plant medicines I was introduced to in my studies within the Wise Woman tradition, my practice of land/place-based herbalism and elemental magic, and my direct education through psilocybin mushrooms, which both my European and Arawak ancestors worked with to access multidimensional spaces of Earth education and healing.

How would you like to see Latine herbalism and curanderismo integrated in our modern age?

I love the new generation of brick-and-mortar *botánicas* (spiritual herb shops) popping up. The feeling is so different from the apothecaries rooted in European herbalism. Both serve people with plants and empower folks through education, but my spirit rejoices to feel more Latine and Afro-Caribbean flavors bringing beauty and diversity to communities in cities across the country. I work with a lot of young Latine, Native, and mixed women who are so sincerely investing in themselves and their communities, dedicated to doing the tender, fierce, ongoing work of reclaiming their roots and culture that were taken and reweaving whole lineages that have been not "lost," as is often said, but disrupted. I think that the more these next generations of healers are supported in healing and reorganizing themselves and taking their places in community, the more wonderful life will be for us all!

Which is your favorite herb, and how do you use it with others and in your personal practice?

Mugwort (*L. Artemisia vulgaris* and *Artemisia douglasiana*) is a favorite that comes to mind. I make bundles that I burn for space clearing, make tea for dream work, and prepare baños with mugwort for more immersive body-based cleansing and to prepare myself to enter ritual spaces.

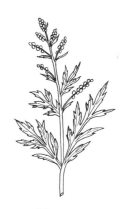

Mugwort

Can you share a simple recipe you love?

Yes! The traditional Puerto Rican diet has been heavily infiltrated by brands that do not have the best interests of the community at heart. I feel very called to the work of figuring out how to re-create my nana's recipes without the use of products that contain artificial flavors, dyes, and other unnecessary nonfood ingredients. Diabetes runs in my family, so I have re-created a familiar flavor from my youth by replacing the commercial guava paste that comes in a can. In this version, I use blood sugar–regulating guava leaf tea and only whole foods. This dish, for me, is healing on so many levels, including bringing back pleasure and sweetness to the embodied experience of being a mixed Boriken/Puerto Rican/Taino American here and now.

Yaya's Blood Sugar–Regulating Herbal Guava Paste Recipe

6 cups water, divided (3 cups cold)

6 tablespoons high-quality gelatin

24 grams (about 12 tea bag) dried guava leaf

1½ cups pink guava powder

9 tablespoons honey

Bloom the gelatin by sprinkling it over 3 cups of cold water in a bowl, stirring continuously to combine. Let stand for 5–10 minutes, until the gelatin has absorbed all the water. This step is important for achieving a smooth texture that is not gritty or lumpy. In a medium saucepan, bring the remaining 3 cups of water to a simmer. Turn off the heat and add the guava leaves. Cover and allow to steep for 5 minutes. Strain into a mixing bowl and whisk in the pink guava powder until it is fully incorporated. Add the bloomed gelatin, whisk together until smooth, and add the honey.

Immediately pour the mixture into a 9 x 11-inch baking pan lined with parchment paper. If your mixture does not appear perfectly smooth, you can pour it into the baking pan through a strainer to remove any remaining gelatin lumps. Cool; refrigerate overnight. Once set, remove the guava paste from the pan by carefully lifting it out by the edges of the parchment paper before slicing it into cubes using a sharp knife.

My nana served guava paste cubes with cheese and crackers, but many Puerto Ricans are gluten and dairy intolerant, as these foods were not part of our traditional diet. I find cashew cheese and almond flour crackers topped with a cube of this herbal guava paste to be irresistibly delicious, and I like to make this recipe for holidays as a way of honoring and giving continuity to our culture without compromising my own best understanding of what serves our health now and going forward.

Contact information: Instagram @medicinariocosmico and @medicinemandala, www.riocosmico.org

NATASHA PACHALOVE

For an immigrant like me, who wasn't raised in one place or even in my ancestral country, community is global. My love for travel and connection encourages me to stay open in anticipation of meeting others who share my interests. But when I meet someone who shares a similar love for the Natural world and is a teacher as well, it bubbles up an emotion I can't describe. When I met Natasha, I felt a connection, and soon enough, I knew we were kindred spirit sisters. I wanted to include her in this book because she carries the energy and knowledge of a curandera. As you will read in the following interview, even the Shipibo elders recognized this. I am also excited to include another Latine from

Borikén. This wonderful island has many riches and is a sister to the Island of Cuba. I can't wait for you to discover more gifts of Las Islas Caribeñas (the Caribbean islands). Natasha holds the beauty of women's traditional health. She supports the rhythm of the cycles from a personal, lived experience.

What is your full name? Include title (if you have one) and whether it is a self- or community-given title.

My birth name is Natasha Joline Naugle Feliciano. The name I work under is Natasha Pachalove, given to me by Madre Ayahuasca in the jungles of el Amazonas (the Amazon) in Pucallpa, Peru. My Taíno name is Gutusúcoku, given to me by Abuela Ana Itzpapalotl Carmona, the founding mother of Danza de la Luna in Borikén. I also carry the title of Reverend Priestess, which I received through my initiation as an ordained minister by the Temple of Isis in Geyserville, California, under the mentorship of master choreographer and Reverend Priestess Anandha Ray.

Where were you born, and where is your Latine heritage from?

I was born in Mayagüez, Borikén. My Latine heritage hails from this island. It is a beautiful blend of our *ancestros Taínos Indígenas* (Indigenous Taíno ancestors) and the African, Spanish, Portuguese, and Italian settlers.

How do you define Latine herbalism, and when were you introduced to it?

I define Latine herbalism as the knowledge and wisdom of the medicinal plants and traditional foods of the lands and territories within Latin America. I define it as a dance of Earth knowledge between the Indigenous peoples of the Americas and the Caribbean along with the African and European influences in these territories. I was first introduced to Latine herbalism in my home, albeit unconsciously. My mother always kept a beautiful ruda (rue) plant growing in the house. I recognized it as important, but I didn't know its purpose. I remember hearing her say that her grandmother, Julia, would make chocolate caliente (hot chocolate) with ruda tea and pair it with Edam *queso de bola* (Edam cheeseball). That was a favorite treat Julia would make for them. That was probably the first time I heard about a plant being used without realizing it had medicinal value.

I was proactively reintroduced to Latine herbalism when I traveled to the jungle in the Peruvian Amazon, to Pucallpa— Shipibo territory. I went to study with a *maestro ayahuascero* (ayahuasca master) in 2016. I engaged in *dietas* (diets), medicinal plant fasting, and connected deeper with la Madre Ayahuasca (Mother Ayahuasca) and the plants my teacher would recommend. We would take walks in the jungle, and he would share with me the different medicinal properties of the plants. They were almost everywhere we looked—hundreds and thousands of plants! This teacher is a seventh-generation Shipibo ayahuascero. His father and his father before him, and the previous five generations, all worked with and recognized the medicinal plants of the jungle. That was when I realized that there is so much more potent healing power in the plants of this Earth than I had previously heard science acknowledge.

Do you have a personal relationship with curanderismo?

I do have a personal relationship with curanderismo, even though I don't use that word to describe the way I work with plants and the healing arts. The first time I heard the word "curandera" was in the jungle with the Shipibo. One of the women, the wife of the ayahuascero I was working with, called me a curandera when she saw me preparing medicine. That was the first time I had ever been called a curandera. I felt shocked and surprised to hear that word. I hold so much respect and honor for that word—I couldn't believe it! I've come to understand curanderismo as a way to practice healing and wellness through plants, energy, ancestral wisdom, and ceremony. Those elements are intricately woven into the way I live my life on a daily basis.

How would you like to see Latine herbalism and curanderismo integrated in our modern age?

I would love to see more young people value the knowledge that our elders carry about medicinal plants and nourishing, whole foods from the Earth. I would love to see consciousness continue to rise as more people remember the healing power of our roots and the medicinal ways of our people. Colonialism has done some powerful work in forcing us to forget who we are; in forcing us to leave our ways and embrace Western medicine and logical thinking in place of intuitive knowing. In curanderismo, our relationship with the plants and how we communicate with them is so essential to how they can heal us and work with us. We get to relate to them in a sacred, respectful, and mutually supportive way. We remember how to tend to them as they tend to us—in body, mind, heart, and spirit. We have to be open to listening to them as we learn to recognize those plants and hear their communication—what plant serves what purpose in each different time of need for ourselves and those we serve. I would love to see more young people interested in and devotedly committed to spending time with elders who carry wisdom about our ancestral and cultural practices with medicinal plants and nourishing food.

Can you share your experience with Latine herbalism as it pertains to women's health?

It is only through rediscovering and remembering my ancestral roots and connection to the medicinal ways of plants and food from the land that I am well today as a Latina woman. I've been a seeker of womb healing for almost ten years, and much of that seeking came from my need to balance my hormones and menstrual cycles. From the time I was very young, I had long moon cycles, usually around sixty days, and once even longer. I had explored Western birth control therapy and many alternative ways of healing, and I explored different holistic healing practices, including Reiki, aromatherapy, and homeopathy. It wasn't until I started therapies with Latine Indigenous roots that I began to see some results—not only physically but also mentally, emotionally, and spiritually. When I started to explore womb massages, baños, and *vapores* (vaginal steam baths), I experienced shorter cycles and felt more hormonal regulation. These womb practices have roots in many different cultures across the Indigenous world.

When I traveled back home to Borikén in 2018, I attended a ceremony with the intention of learning where I needed to be and what I needed to do in order to fulfill my purpose. I had become more familiar with plants from the West Coast, like yarrow, sage, and lavender, because I was living in California at the time. Coming to that ceremony back home in Puerto Rico helped me meet so many others who had knowledge of these plants that I didn't yet know but felt in my heart were all I needed to be well and thrive in this life. After the ceremony, I received a clear message from the whispers of the grandmothers of my matriarchal line. They were telling me, through the vibrations I felt from the Earth through the bottoms of my feet, that I needed to be on that land, my motherland of Borikén, to live my purpose. It was then that I started to connect more deeply with *orégano brujo* (Cuban oregano), *ortiga brava* (giant stinging nettle), romero (rosemary), and *poleo* (pennyroyal). Bit by bit, these plants helped me ground into this beautiful body. They helped me channel my creative force for what I was designed to give and receive.

What is the number-one herb for a happy, healthy woman?

The number-one herb for a happy, healthy woman is the herb that the women in her family lineage have worked with ancestrally—the herb she feels most connected to on the land she lives on. Many grandmothers have told me that the plants that grow around you are the ones that have medicine for you. My recommendation is to do research and ask your mother and grandmother, if you still have a connection with them. Ask them if they remember any plants that the women in their family have worked with. If you live on land that's different from your ancestral homelands, talk to the original people about the land and see what herbs are used for optimal women's health there. For example, in Oregon, one might work with mugwort; in California, one might work with yarrow.

Here in Borikén, my number-one herb for a happy, healthy woman is *ortiga brava* (giant stinging nettle). This variety is botanically different from the small-leaved stinging nettle found up north, although many of the properties are similar. It is an herb I use myself and recommend. If you come into contact with it, approach it with respect. Handle with gloves until ready to use and keep away from children. It's wonderful for circulation, regulating hormones, hair growth, and all-around vitality. For me, it was the first plant I deeply connected to after moving back to the island. I began to take tinctures of ortiga brava on a daily basis. This tincture helped regulate my cycle for the first time in my life. I finally felt like I was in balance; I finally felt strong and vital in my body and that my internal fire was lit, ready to create.

Can you share a recipe with a favorite herb?

You can take ortiga brava or any stinging nettle variety in the form of a *guarapo*—our traditional *jíbaro* (traditional farmer) term on the island for making a water extraction or medicinal tea with the plant's stems, roots, and tougher leathery leaves.

For this recipe, I want to give thanks to María Benedetti, an incredible herbal teacher, for rescuing and remembering our traditional medicinal plants on the island of Borikén. Through her work, María interviewed jíbaro elders from the mountainous countryside and documented their oral histories in *Earth and Spirit: Medicinal Plants and Healing Lore from Puerto Rico* (1989) and other books, which explore and celebrate Puerto Rico's tradition of botanical medicine as it was practiced up to the 1980s.

Hormone Balancing Nettle Tea Recipe

Giant stinging nettle (*L. Urera baccifera*)—*Ortiga brava*
Stinging nettle (*L. Urtica*)—*Ortiga mayor*

ENERGY: Hot/dry | TASTE: Bitter/salty/mineral | PLANT PARTS
USED: Leaf

> 3–4 cups water
> handful of ortiga brava leaves or available nettle family
> mason jar

Bring the water to a boil, add the ortiga leaves, and
simmer for 10–25 minutes. Strain and drink warm in the
evening.

Nettle

Tincture option: You can make the nettle into a
tincture for greater accessibility and consumption.
Fill the mason jar with dried or fresh ortiga, pack it
down tightly, and top off the jar with your alcohol of
choice. You can use rum, or here on the island, we
sometimes use *pitorro* (Puerto Rican moonshine). Cover with a
lid and let it sit for six weeks, shaking it with love and intention
once a day. After this period, the tincture can be strained and
stored in colored glass bottles. Take by the dropper as needed.

Remedio option: Another way to use ortiga brava, and my
favorite, most effective method, is to use the fresh leaf for an
ortigazo—a term referring to the stinging action of the nettle that
is a portmanteau of "ortiga" and "*punzón*" (sting). Rosita, an elder
herbalist here in Moca, taught me this remedio as it is always done
with an experienced practioner. You take the fresh leaf harvested
straight from the plant and place it on the body. The spikes of the
leaf bring relief from inflammation, allowing the stinging action
of the ortiga to promote blood flow. If my moon cycle feels late
and I sense heaviness in my womb, I will take the fresh leaf and
press it onto my lower abdomen to activate circulation while

I breathe deeply into the stinging, warming sensation to bring release.

Contact information: Instagram @natashapachalove www.thesacredremembrance.com

ROSA MAYA

As an educator and lover of cacao, I visited Guatemala in 2024 to learn more about the Maya lineages of Cacao. I had the pleasure of meeting Rosa Maya, a traditional herbalist and someone I consider so intertwined with the land that her knowledge has no category. While she works specifically with Mayan abdominal massage, I found my *temazcalli* (temazcal treatment) experience with her to be transformational. Here was this tiny woman who turned into a lioness in the womb of the Mother! I am not easily impressed, but that day in the *temazcal* (Indigenous sweat lodge) at the edge of Lake Atitlán, I knew I had met someone very special. Even her writing holds a certain poetic, ephemeral energy.

The temazcal is important in many cultures, not just as a healing space but as a community space. *Temazcales* appear in Teotihuacán frescoes dating back to Mesoamerican times that portray communal baths and the use of *vapores*. It is an important ritual in Mexican curanderismo and was the one missing part of sharing Latine herbalism with you all, as temazcal is used as a healing modality all over Latin America specially for postpartum health. I am thrilled that you can read the teachings of temazcalli from one of my teachers. The original Spanish follows the English interview. Rosa Maya holds the lineages of Cacao, Temazcal, and Mayan womb healing. I hope to return to Guatemala and continue my studies with her—maybe you can join us!

Where were you born, and where is your Latine heritage from?

I was born in Boyacá in the Colombian Andes, where my grandmothers saw me grow up, and with their love and wisdom of plants and good food, they raised me.

How do you define Latine herbalism?

Traditional medicine does not have written pages; everything is oral and learned through practice. I grew up learning about herbs alongside the herbs and herbal baths.

When were you introduced to Latine herbalism?

Herbalism is very wild where I grew up, and you learn to recognize it when you are a small child. For as long as I can remember, I have been introduced to herbalism. Growing up, we did not use medicines. I wasn't sickly as a child either, so there was no need for doctors. We didn't have money for expensive treatments and learned to take care of ourselves with hierbitas.

Do you have a personal relationship with curanderismo?

"Curanderismo" is a very big word. In our pueblos, we knew of hueseros, *sobadores* (masseuses), and curanderas, but they were not called curanderas/os. They are called by their names, without titles. There are not many left in the pueblos; many have migrated to the big cities or abroad. Medicine is no longer practiced. They carry it inside to the Western world and follow the American dream. But like you and me, we carry it inside until the magic awakens.

Do you have a favorite herb?

I have many plants that guide me and that grow in my garden. I don't have a favorite;—I have many, hahaha! As a Medicine Woman, I have seasonal herbs and herbs that are good for me. It depends on what is around you. Right now, I am a big fan of lemon verbena. Since childhood, I have known calendula, yarrow, rue, rosemary, rose, sage, and endless plants.

Where did you learn about the temazcal and its healing properties?

The temazcal was one of the medicines that awakened me, and I thank the Medicine Women of Mexico for this gift. I learned about temazcal from a Mexican grandmother in Oaxaca, Mexico. She was subtle and profound. This woman and many others taught me during that time. I gave myself without knowing that one day I would hold the healing spaces of temazcales.

As a *temazcalera* (practitioner of temazcal), what is your view of this ancestral practice as it applies to wellness today?

The temazcal is an ancestral bath of Abya Yala, the Americas; the ancestral Grandparents throughout America had a form of temazcal, Inipi, sweatlodge, etc. It is the Momb of Mother Earth, where we can undress without any fear. Where the Grandfather and Grandmother Elements speak to us and listen to our pleas. The Grandmother stones have to be volcanic rock containing pure minerals. They can also be from the river but the Temazcalero knows to be careful.

It is a ceremony. There are many rituals and ways to hold healing space in a temazcalli. The grandmothers and grandfathers and the four directions are invoked. Blessings and permission are requested from the land where you are holding this ritual, and here begins all the mystery and healing. Medicine songs are part of the ritual, as in all ancestral rituals of the Americas. These help transform and quiet the mind. There needs to be a lot of respect for all the medicines of the world. I know that today the temazcalli is very popular, and it has become an experience, but people don't benefit from this experience just because they can pay for it.

It is important to have an intention in a temazcalli ritual. The elemental grandparents are burning for you. Wood, water, and the Temazcalero form a channel for your transformation and pleas. The temazcalli centers around Grandfather Fire. I work with my plants also. I know they can help people; the steam bath I offer is therapeutic.

As the grandmothers taught me, I offer the temazcalli and live up to their teaching ways with all my love and respect. I continue to learn more about temazcales from grandmothers and grandfathers—resting the body and soul to continue to be of service; making my pilgrimages, my sacrifices, and fasts to prepare further.

Grateful to be able to enter Mother's womb, where she receives us, where she cuddles us and listens to us, where the fire sears us until the wind is transformed into song and the Earth sustains our songs and cries. It is there that Mama Temazcalli opens the doors of her heart so we can pray near the elemental grandmothers. A pleasure that you can read my words.

Contact information: Instagram @raizdulce

The interview in Spanish:

¿Dónde naciste y de dónde es tu herencia Latina?

Nací en los Andes Colombianos Boyacá Aquí mis abuelas me vieron crecer y, con su amor, sabiduría de plantas y buen alimento, me criaron.

¿Cómo defines la herbolaria Latina?

La medicina tradicional no tiene hojas escritas, todo es oral y en práctica. Crecí tomando herbolaria al lado de las plantas y los baños de herbolaria.

¿Cuándo fuiste introducida a la herbolaria Latina?

Es muy silvestre la herbolaria por mi territorio y aprendes a conocerla cuando estás pequeño. Desde que tengo memoria, fui introducida a la herbolaria. En mis tiempos, no usaba medicamentos. No fui una niña tan enferma como para los médicos. No disponíamos de dinero para tratamientos caros, así que nos cuidamos.

¿Tienes una relación con el curanderismo?

"Curanderismo" es una palabra muy grande. En nuestros pueblos solían haber hueseros, sobadores y curanderas, pero no se llamaban curanderas/os. Se les llama por su nombre. Pues ahora ya no hay muchos en los pueblos, en unas épocas migraron a la ciudad y exterior, ya no se practicaba la medicina. La llevan dentro, pero por el mundo occidental y el "sueño americano" se fueron perdiendo. Pero, así como tú y yo, lo llevamos dentro y surge el despertar de esta magia.

¿Tienes una hierba favorita?

Tengo muchas plantas que me guían y que tengo en mi jardín. No tengo una favorita—tengo muchas jajaja! Como Mujer Medicina, tengo las de la temporada y las que me hacen bien. Depende de lo que tengas. Ahora soy muy fan del cedrón, pero desde niña conozco la caléndula, milenrama, ruda, romero, rosa, salvia, bueno, un sinfín de plantas.

¿Dónde aprendiste del temazcal y sus propiedades curativas?

El temazcal fue una de las medicinas que me ayudó a despertar, y le agradezco a las Mujeres Medicina de México. Lo conocí con una abuela mexicana en Oaxaca, tan sutil, tan profunda. Esta mujer y otras más que tuve en ese momento a mi alrededor me enseñaron; me entregué sin saber que algún día correría temazcales.

Como una temazcalera, ¿cómo referencias esta práctica ancestral para aplicarla al dÌa de hoy e incluirla al concepto de bienestar moderno?

El temazcal es un baño ancestral de Abya Yala (las américas). Los abuelos caminantes en todo américa tenían su temazcal, inípi, etc. Es el vientre de Madre Tierra, allí donde nos podemos desnudar sin miedo alguno. Donde los abuelos y abuelas elementos nos hablan, nos escuchan. Las abuelas piedras tienen que ser volcánicas; tienen minerales puros. También pueden ser de río, pero el que corre temazcales sabe que hay que tener cuidado.

Es una ceremonia. Hay muchos rituales y formas de correr un temazcalli. Se invocan los y las abuelas y las cuatro direcciones. Se pide permiso al territorio donde estás y allí empieza todo el misterio y la sanación. Los cantos, como en toda América, son parte del ritual. Ayudan a transformar y aquietar la mente. Hay que tener mucho respeto con todas las medicinas del mundo y respetar. Sé que ahora el temazcal es muy famoso y se volvió una experiencia. Peor a la gente no les ayuda solo tener la experiencia y pagar por ella.

Es importante tener un propósito, porque allí se están quemando los abuelos por ti. La madera, el agua y la persona que guía es un canal para ayudarte en tu transformación, petición. Aquí todo es con el abuelo fuego. por lo general entro mis plantas que sé que ayudan a las personas; el baño de vapor que yo hago es terapéutico.

Así como las abuelas me transmitieron así lo llevo, con todo mi amor y respeto. Recibiendo temazcales de abuelas y abuelos, yendo a descansar el ser para poder ofrecer este servicio. Haciendo mis peregrinaciones, mis pagamentos y mis ayunos. Agradecida por poder entrar al vientre de Mamá, allí donde mamita nos recibe, allí donde nos arrulla y nos escucha, y el fuego nos abrasa tanto que el viento se transforma en canto. La tierra nos sostiene el canto y el llanto. Es allí donde Mamá Temazcalli nos abre las puertas de su corazón para rezar cerca de los y las abuelas Elementales. Un gusto que puedan leerme.

IAN DARRAH

Ian is one of the first yoga teachers I met in Miami. We had realized we had a lot in common when we had the opportunity to chat about yoga and shamanism. Hc is one of the few practitioners of shamanic Indigenous practices that works from the heart. Unlike many centers and people in the USA, Ian is very particular in the context of healing with master plants. In addition to valuing his twenty years of experience, I trust only him when the need of these practices arrises. As a French American man, his view was important to include in this book. Latine herbalism and curanderismo is not just for those of Latine culture and background. The healing arts of Latin America are open to all, especially when used with reverence and love. Ian exemplifies this. His wife Gaby, whom he met in Peru, has many times mentioned that when Ian works with master plants, he transforms into a curandero and is physically unrecognizable. I have seen him myself and recognize the Espiritu of the Amazon in him. It is an honor to call him my friend and to share with you his words.

What is your full name, include title (If you have one) and if it is a self- or community-given title?

Ian "Ram Dass" Darrah, a mentor and teacher of Yoga Philosophy and the healing traditions of the Americas.

I have mentored thousands of students for more than twenty years, and widely recognized as a knowledgeable and powerful carrier of the wisdom traditions.

Teaching from experience of decades as an impassioned student of health, longevity, human potential, and daily dedication to personal development and the empowerment of others.

My title was given by Swami Brahma Vidyananda of the Satyananda/Bihar School.

Can you share a little about your background?

My maternal cultural lineage is French, my paternal lineage is American (Welsh, Dutch, German) but I've dedicated my life to sharing yoga and meditation, blessed by a traditional Swami in the Sivananda-Satyananda lineage.

For the past twenty years I've also been deeply transformed by Master Plant Medicine Ceremonies and sacred rituals like Sweat Lodge, Vision Quest, Sun Dance, and shamanic/Indigenous rituals. These experiences have profoundly enhanced my teaching, allowing me to guide others more intuitively and in a deeper, more effective way.

When did you become interested in Latine herbalism and curandersimo?

Ever since I was a child I was fascinating by the way of life of the North American Indians and Indigenous people. As a teenager, I read about Latine sacred master plant use in certain rituals and was deeply intrigued.

What is your relationship to curandersimo and shamanism, how do these two modalities interweave in your experience?

My relationship with curanderismo and shamanism is deeply rooted in a profound spiritual journey that began over twenty years ago when I took my first yoga class. From that moment, I encountered a level of healing, health, and therapeutic access that resonated within me on a soul-deep level. I remember lying in savasana (relaxation pose) for the first time in my life with a smile on my face knowing that every atom and cell in my body were saying "follow this path!" It was as if I had rediscovered a vital part of myself, and I felt an unshakeable conviction in my heart that I would embark on the path of yoga and meditation for a lifetime. Little did I know, this initial step onto the mat would open a doorway to a broader exploration of spiritual modalities.

Around the same time, my journey took me to Brazil, where I became immersed in Indigenous American Shamanic practices that would further shape my understanding of healing and spiritual connection. Participating in a Vision Quest, engaging in ayahuasca and peyote master plant medicine ceremonies, enduring sweat lodges, and supporting the Mexican Sun Dance were experiences that catalyzed a profound transformation within me. Each of these rituals and ceremonies brought with it layers of healing, introspection, and connection to something greater than the story I had in my mind about myself. The experiences defied conventional description; they were spiritual and mystical, rich in metaphor, visions, and insights that felt beyond the reach of everyday language. I often found myself grappling with the weight of what I had witnessed—a reality that many people on this planet may never encounter in their lifetime.

Initially, I perceived the yoga/meditation path and the shamanic plant medicine paths as starkly different. Yoga, with its emphasis on mindfulness, breath, and the alignment of mind, body, and spirit, seemed distinct from the more ancestral, earth-based practices of shamanism that engaged directly with the spirit world and plant allies. However, as years passed, my perspectives evolved, and I began to recognize the intricate ways these seemingly divergent paths intertwine, creating a rich tapestry of healing and awakening. I even discovered that many fundamental principles and outcomes of the main practices in each of these paths were the same. This was an epiphany.

What I realized is that beneath their differing external appearances lies a common objective: the quest for holistic healing and self-realization. Yoga aims to harmonize the physical, emotional, and spiritual aspects of the self, leading practitioners toward a deeper sense of inner peace, unity, connection, consciousness, and understanding. Similarly, the shamanic practices call upon ancient wisdom and connection with nature to facilitate healing and transformation. At their core, both modalities tap into the same internal mechanisms and processes of the mind-body-spirit triad, allowing us, through purification, to access profound states of awareness and connection.

Through my journey, I've come to appreciate how both practices can complement one another. The disciplined practice of yoga enhances my awareness and prepares my body and mind for the deeper, often more intense experiences found in shamanic rituals. In turn, the insights gained from shamanic experiences enrich my yoga practice, deepening my understanding of energy flow and spiritual connection. I see this synthesis as a powerful reminder that healing and spirituality can take many forms, and ultimately, they lead us toward the same destination: unity, love, and the sacredness of all life.

How would you like to see curanderismo and shamanism integrated in this modern age?

In envisioning the integration of curanderismo and shamanism in today's world, it is essential to emphasize the deep-rooted principles that these traditions embody—principles that honor ancestral wisdom and the time-honored medicinal practices that have been passed down through generations. Curanderismo, at its core, is not just a set of techniques or a methodology; it is a holistic system that calls us to remember and connect with the healing practices that have nourished and sustained Indigenous and tribal peoples for millennia—a living tradition that gets channeled and transmitted. It is fundamentally about honoring the knowledge that has been cultivated over time, from the wise ones of the past, and recognizing the profound relationship between the modern individual and the natural world.

This path involves a systemic body of knowledge rooted in the life-affirming and health-enhancing properties of plants, elements, and nature itself. A true "curanderas/o" embodies this wisdom through direct experience, engaging with the plants and other natural remedies first on a personal level before offering support to others. This intimate relationship is cultivated slowly, often over many years, and is characterized by a depth of understanding that transcends book knowledge. In essence, the work of a curanderas/o is an embodied practice rather than a theoretical one.

In our fast-paced modern society, where many seek quick answers through digital means—Google serving as a modern oracle—there exists a challenge to the authentic flow of healing that curanderismo offers. The essence of natural healing is rooted in experience, relationship, and presence, rather than mere information transfer. A true curandera/o communes with the living energy of plants, minerals, animals, and the elements, developing a deep wisdom and understanding through personal experience that informs their healing practices. This experiential wisdom cannot be captured in a book.

As we navigate the complexities of modern life, many people find themselves yearning for immediate fixes and succinct answers to their ailments, often overlooking the inherent complexities involved in the holistic healing process. This urgency can result in a diminished understanding of the patience and dedication required to engage genuinely in the healing journey.

Recognizing this gap, I believe that many curanderas/os today are stepping into the pivotal role of educators as well as healers. They are taking on the important responsibility of guiding those in need of healing while also cultivating a deeper understanding and appreciation for what natural healing truly entails. Through workshops, community ceremonies, and shared experiences, curanderas/os can bridge the gap between ancient wisdom and contemporary needs, allowing individuals to reconnect with the land, their heritage, and their own bodies.

In this modern age, I envision a harmonious blending of traditional practices like curanderismo and shamanism, with contemporary healing principles, where education plays a vital role in both demystifying natural healing and honoring the inherent magic and mystery (the mystical) at the same time!

Do you have a favorite herb, and how do you use it with others and in your personal practice for yourself?

Among the vast array of herbs and superfoods that nurture my body and soul, my heart belongs to the revered Plantas Maestras, "Master Teacher Plants." These potent botanicals—ayahuasca, huachuma, psilocybin mushrooms, peyote, and iboga—have been transformative gifts from Nature's apothecary, guided by the loving hands of skilled curanderos. These sacred medicines have unraveled the intricacies of my being, revealing hidden truths and healing the trifecta of mind, body, and spirit.

Huachuma, the majestic San Pedro, holds a special place in my personal practice. This ancient plant ally whispers secrets of the heart, encouraging me to listen to the subtle rhythms of my inner world. With reverence, I prepare the medicine, boiling and straining its essence for hours, infused with mantras, chants, and the sacred mapacho blessings. My beloved wife's presence bears witness to this ritual, as we cocreate a sanctuary for spiritual growth.

In micro-doses, huachuma becomes an intimate companion, guiding me through the labyrinth of my inner space. I attune to the harmonics of my living environment, seeking balance between the inner and outer worlds. On select days, I commit to a deeper journey, surrendering to the medicine's twelve-hour odyssey. As the entheogenic effects unfold, my body becomes a canvas of sensation, revealing areas of blockage and trauma. The Sushumna nadis, the ethereal pathway of my spinal cord, stir, and my low back, scarred from past injuries, trembles. Tears flow like autumn rain as frozen memories thaw, releasing the weight of yesterday.

The aftermath of these journeys beckons rest, a surrender to the void, allowing the wisdom to integrate, like the gentle rainfall nourishing the parched earth.

As a master practitioner, I approach these medicines with reverence and caution, recognizing their potency. My twenty years of experience have taught me the importance of surrender, trust, and self-awareness when venturing into the depths of the psychedelic experience.

In the stillness, I acknowledge the power of these Master Teacher Plants, humble guardians of ancient wisdom. They remind me that the true magic lies not in the plants themselves, but in the sacred relationship between the plant, the healer, and the seeker. May their wisdom continue to guide me on my journey, and may I honor their potency with reverence and care.

Can you share a practice for wellness in these modern times?

For me, yoga is the pinnacle of wellness practices. To experience its transformative power, find a local class and teacher who inspires you. Make yoga a habit, and watch yourself grow. Ideally, find a studio with a nurturing community that fosters connection and support. And, even better, you can supercharge your wellness practice by getting more in tune and connected with the plants. Some traditional Indian Yoga Ashrams, for example, recommend before starting your yoga practice to have some neem and turmeric with a bit of warm water. Others might recommend a bit of tulsi tea with some ginger and honey. I feel a synergy of body and mind when I practice yoga that incorporate the use of these herbs.

Yoga is especially vital in modern times, where sedentary lifestyles pose the greatest health risk. Regular movement is essential. Supplement your yoga practice with daily walks or jogs. To amplify the benefits, incorporate this simple yet profound breath exercise into your walks or jogs:

- Inhale for 4 steps
- Hold breath for 4 steps
- Exhale for 4 steps
- Hold again for 4 steps
  Repeat for 10–20 minutes, harmonizing breath and movement. This yogic technique, known as pranayama, calms the mind, balances the body, and cultivates

mindfulness. By embracing yoga, medicinal herbs, and conscious movement, you'll unlock a life-changing journey toward holistic wellness.

Contact information: Instagram @iandarrah_ramdass www.iandarrahyoga.com

RESOURCES

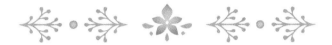

The best place to shop is in your neighborhood herb shops and botánicas, community apothecaries, and local farmers markets. But if you need to purchase plant materials and ritual supplies online, try these options:

- MountainRoseHerbs.com—Mountain Rose Herbs carries sustainable, ethically sourced herbs and spices.
- EdenBotanicals.com—Eden Botanicals offers essential oils, carrier oils, and hard-to-find apothecary materials from around the world.
- NewDirectionsAromatics.com—New Directions Aromatics carries a large selection of organic oils, herbs, and candle and soap-making supplies.
- WellingtonFragrance.com—Wellington Fragrance delivers premium fragrance oils, carrier oils, and essential oils for all apothecary recipes.
- BulkApothecary.com—Bulk Apothecary specializes in organic oils and hard-to-find oils for apothecary and soap making.

- BanyanBotanicals.com—Banyan Botanicals is an Ayurveda-centered shop offering herbs, liquid extracts, and specialty infused oils.
- CuranderaRemedies.com—Curandera Remedies is an indie brand offering ritual supplies along with online curanderismo courses and personalized sessions.
- LatineHerbalism.com—The Latine Herbalism website brings this book to life. Find apothecary kits, herbalism courses, and retreats to further your studies in Latine herbalism.
- LosCavazosTexas.com—Los Cavazos Texas offers Mexican herbs and blends for teas, tinctures, and other apothecary items.

You can find many apothcary-making materials from neighborhood stores and big-name retailers such as Walmart, Amazon, and Ebay.

REFERENCES

Avila, Elena, with Joy Parker. *Woman Who Glows in the Dark: A Curandera Reveals Traditional Aztec Secrets of Physical and Spiritual Health*. TarcherPerigee, 2000.

Ávila, Mary Carmen M. "Levantada de Cruz, su significado ante la muerte de un ser querido." *El Sol de Puebla,* March 23, 2023. https://www.elsoldepuebla.com.mx/cultura/levantada-de-cruz -su-significado-ante-la-muerte-de-un-ser-querido-9807109.html.

Benedetti, María. *Earth and Spirit: Medicinal Plants and Healing Lore from Puerto Rico*. Waterfront Press, 1989. Reprint, Verde Luz, 1998.

Blaser, Janet. "Understanding Canela, or Mexican Cinnamon." *Mexico News Daily,* October 16, 2021. https://mexiconewsdaily.com /mexico-living/understanding-canela-or-mexican-cinnamon.

Brennan, Barbara Ann. *Hands of Light: A Guide to Healing Through the Human Energy Field*. Bantam, 1988.

Biblioteca Digital de la Medicina Tradicional Mexicana. "Levantar la Sombra." http://www.medicinatradicionalmexicana.unam.mx /demtm/termino.php?l=1&t=levantar-sombra.

Botanical Revival. "Linden Monograph: For When You Just Need a Friend," March 30, 2023. https://botanicalrevivalherbs.com /linden-monograph.

Buenaflor, Erika. *Cleansing Rites of Curanderismo: Limpias Espirituales of Ancient Mesoamerican Shamans.* Bear & Company, 2018.

Tonic: Therapeutic Herb Shop and Elixir Bar. "Cacao." https:// tonicherbshop.com/cacao.

Cambron, Melisa. "A Comparison of Historical and Current Use of Salvia Divinorum in the United States and Mexico." *Lake Forest College—Department of Biology*, February 26, 2016. https:// www.lakeforest.edu/news/a-comparison-of-historical-and-current -use-of-salvia-divinorum-in-the-united-states-and-mexico.

Castledine, David B., trans. *Popol Vuh: The Sacred Book of the Ancient Mayas-Quiché.* Monclem Ediciones, 2001.

Emoto, Masaru. *The Hidden Messages in Water.* Atria Books, 2005.

"El empacho: Una enfermedad popular Latinoamericana." *Cuadernos de Historia de la Salud Pública* (Havana) 102 (July–December 2007). http://scielo.sld.cu/scielo.php?script=sci_arttext&pid =S0045-91782007000200004.

Getty Research Institute. "Through the Obsidian Mirror." *Obsidian Mirror-Travels*, November 16, 2010. https:// www.getty.edu/research/exhibitions_events/exhibitions/obsidian _mirror/through_the_mirror.html.

Graves, Julia. *The Language of Plants: A Guide to the Doctrine of Signatures.* Lindisfarne Books, 2012.

iNaturalistMX. "Artemisa." https://mexico.inaturalist.org/taxa /52856-Artemisia-vulgaris.

Mendoza Nunziato, Rebecca. "Sacred Smoke of Copal: From Mesoamerican Religion to Chicanx Ceremonies." *ReVista (Harvard Review of Latin America)*, February 22, 2021. https:// revista.drclas.harvard.edu/sacred-smoke-of-copal.

NASA Science Mission Directorate. "Anatomy of an Electromagnetic Wave." *NASA Science*, 2010. https://science.nasa.gov/ems /02_anatomy.

Nassau, Kurt. "The Visible Spectrum." *Britannica.* Last updated October 21, 2024. https://www.britannica.com/science/color /The-visible-spectrum.

Nunez, Kristen. "What Is Palo Santo, and How Is It Used Medicinally?" *Healthline,* August 11, 2020. https:// www.healthline.com/health/palo-santo-benefits.

Pérez Campa, Mario, and Laura Sotelo Santos. *The Mayas: The Splendor of a Great Culture.* Monclem Ediciones, 2006.

Quiñonez-Bastidas GN, Navarrete A. "Mexican Plants and Derivates Compounds as Alternative for Inflammatory and Neuropathic Pain Treatment-A Review." National Library of Medicine, April 25, 2021 https://pmc.ncbi.nlm.nih.gov/articles/PMC8145628.

Research Gate. "Ethnobotany of Medicinal Flora in Two Communities of the Mixteca Alta in Oaxaca, Mexico," May 2020. https:// www.researchgate.net/publication/362777641_ETHNOBOTANY _OF_MEDICINAL_FLORA_IN_TWO_COMMUNITIES_OF _THE_MIXTECA_ALTA_IN_OAXACA_MEXICO _ETNOBOTANICA_DE_LA_FLORA_MEDICINAL_EN_DOS _COMUNIDADES.

Romero-Cerecero, Ofelia, Alejandro Zamilpa-Álvarez, Enrique Jiménez-Ferrer, and Jaime Tortoriello. "Exploratory Study on the Effectiveness of a Standardized Extract from Ageratina Pichinchensis in Patients with Chronic Venous Leg Ulcers." *Planta Medica* 78, no. 4 (2012): 304–10. https://pubmed.ncbi.nlm.nih.gov /22174074.

Torres, Axel. "La herbolaria, medicina antigua y tradicional." *Gaceta,* December 4, 2020. https://gaceta.facmed.unam.mx/index.php /2020/12/04/la-herbolaria-medicina-antigua-y-tradicional.

Torres, Eliseo "Cheo." *Healing with Herbs and Rituals: A Mexican Tradition.* University of New Mexico Press, 2006.

Torres, Eliseo "Cheo," and Imanol Miranda. *Curandero: Traditional Healers of Mexico and the Southwest.* Kendall Hunt, 2017.

Trotter II, Robert T., and Juan Antonio Chavira. *Curanderismo: Mexican American Folk Healing.* 2nd ed. University of Georgia Press, 1997.

Wood, Matthew. *The Practice of Traditional Western Herbalism: Basic Doctrine, Energetics, and Classification.* North Atlantic Books, 2004.

Zavaleta, Antonio Noé. *Curandero: Hispanic Ethno-Psychotherapy and Curanderismo—Treating Hispanic Mental Health in the 21st Century.* AuthorHouse, 2020.

ACKNOWLEDGMENTS

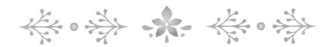

I am forever grateful to the ones who came before me—the ancestors whom I never met but whose knowledge is braided into my bones. I am also in deep gratitude to my mother, Candelaria Castañeda, and father, Leo Castañeda, who instilled in me a love and pride in my heritage and culture.

This book and its contents would not have manifested if I had not met Julia Graves. Without her guidance during the earlier days in my studies, I would not have the clarity, focus, and determination to dive deep into the healing arts and find my path as a yerbera curandera. Thank you Julia!

Un millón de gracias to my friends and family, who with patience and joy supported the creation of this book. Special thanks to Yaya Erin, Natasha Pachamama, Rosa Maya, and Iansito: gracias, gracias, gracias!!

Lastly, I bow at the feet of the Goddess Lalita. The great Maha Shakti, I am, because She is. *Jai ma*!

ABOUT THE AUTHOR

Iosellev "Josie" Castañeda Morales is a modern-day curandera. At an early age she was introduced to the practice of curanderismo as a way of life. Today, Josie serves her Miami community as a yerbera, one who works with herbs. She shares her knowledge with depth, joy, and clarity. You can connect with her at CuranderaRemedies.com.